D0875453

A Step-by-Step Guide to Dealing With Your Breast Cancer

A Step-by-Step Guide to Dealing With Your Breast Cancer

Rebecca Y. Robinson
and
Jeanne A. Petrek, M.D.

A BIRCH LANE PRESS BOOK

Published by Carol Publishing Group

A Birch Lane Press Book
Published by Carol Publishing Group
Birch Lane Press is a registered trademark of Carol Communications, Inc.
Editorial Offices: 600 Madison Avenue, New York, N.Y. 10022
Sales and Distribution Offices: 120 Enterprises Avenue, Secaucus, N.J. 07094
In Canada: Canadian Manda Group, P.O. Box 920, Station U, Toronto, Ontario M8Z 5P9
Queries regarding rights and permissions should be addressed to Carol Publishing Group, 600 Madison Avenue, New York, N.Y. 10022

Carol Publishing Group books are available at special discounts for bulk purchases, sales promotions, fund-raising, or educational purposes. Special editions can be created to specifications. For details, contact Special Sales Department, Carol Publishing Group, 120 Enterprise Avenue, Secaucus, N.J. 07094

Manufactured in the United States of America

10 9 8 7 6 5 4 3 2 1

Library of Congress Cataloging-in-Publication Data

Robinson, Rebecca Y.
  A step-by-step guide to dealing with your breast cancer /
by Rebecca Y. Robinson and Jeanne A. Petrek.
      p.   cm.
  "A Birch Lane Press book."
  ISBN 1-55972-257-6
  1. Breast—Cancer—Popular works. I. Petrek, Jeanne A.
II. Title
RC280.B8R588   1994
616.99'449—dc20   94-18102
                                                       CIP

Contents

Part Four
The Real Costs: Emotional and Financial

Part Five
A Database of Sources and Resources

Acknowledgments

For Suzanne, and all women who have had breast cancer, we salute your courage. We appreciate your willingness to help others with their breast cancer diagnoses. We commend you for your diligence in working with doctors in pursuit of better care. We applaud your activism in bringing the issue to those who are in a position to legislate and financially support the challenge to find a cure.

We want to give our sincere gratitude to Loretta Barrett for her confidence in this project and her editorial support in the "journey" to publication. And, our thanks to Hillel Black for his sound editorial advice and genuine interest in breast cancer.

Introduction

Dr. Petrek and I have written *A Step-by-Step Guide to Dealing With Your Breast Cancer* for the millions of American women who live with breast cancer either through anticipation, suspicion, or reality. It has been estimated by the National Breast Cancer Coalition that 2.6 million women in the United States are living with breast cancer, 1.6 million who have been diagnosed and in treatment for breast cancer, and 1 million who do not yet know that they have breast cancer. Do we anticipate getting breast cancer? Not really, but we know we could develop it and that alone places breast cancer near the top of any woman's list of fears. It is now, and will be, the most discussed and dreaded disease for us in the 1990s. When I first discovered a lump in my breast, all those fears and suspicions surfaced. I thought about cancer and the quality of my life; I thought about mastectomy and losing my breast, or worse, dying. I thought about how my husband, family, and friends would react to the knowledge that I might have breast cancer. Finally, and ultimately, I wondered how I was going to get through what would be an ugly reality.

The idea of writing a book about my experience with breast cancer did not immediately occur to me, even though many other women have done so. Frankly, during the year that it took from the discovery of a suspicious lump in my breast until completing my last chemotherapy treatment, I was totally preoccupied with getting the best possible treatment for my breast cancer.

During that year, and since completing treatment, I did not hide the fact that I had breast cancer. In fact, I have been openly vocal about it. I have met with other breast cancer patients at support groups and lectures; I speak with doctors, like Dr. Petrek, who are specialists in treating breast cancer. I have been to Washington to learn more about breast cancer legislation. I speak with insurance companies and their representatives regarding coverage after cancer. I attend seminars and focus groups for breast cancer updates at regional and urban hospitals and I volunteer for the American Cancer Society.

As a result, I have spoken with women from all over the United States about their need for concrete information about breast cancer, either for themselves or a family member, a relative, or a friend. Some of the women were patients currently in treatment for breast cancer, but most with whom I spoke have had the disease. Other women with significant family histories of cancer were also concerned about the issue.

From my discussions with them, what came through loud and clear were the problems on how to handle the diagnosis. The majority of women felt that they needed advice on how to proceed in getting that first suspicious lump diagnosed, what that diagnosis meant in terms of choosing treatment options, and what they needed to know and do to connect and communicate with the hospitals and specialists that could help cure them. Clearly there was a need for a book on managing the diagnosis of breast cancer.

In trying to piece together the important elements of a useful book, I recalled my own struggle to confirm my breast cancer diagnosis and to investigate my treatment options. It became clear to me in my research that for many women one of the most troubling aspects of breast cancer was dealing with the mechanics of the diagnosis. As problems and uncertainties surfaced from discussions with other breast cancer patients, I had a shopping list of questions regarding the diagnosis.

I knew I could write on my own experience and on the experiences of other women who have had breast cancer, but that would only be half of the picture. What I needed was a medical professional who would not only respond to my questions, but who would provide the rationale of managing the disease from a medical perspective. Dr. Jeanne Petrek, a specialist in breast cancer research and treatment, agreed with the concept of an informative book by doctor and patient. She brings the breadth and depth of her expertise to clarify the diagnostic process.

Our goal in writing *A Step-by-Step Guide to Dealing With Your Breast Cancer* is to provide a first-person, candid, systematic approach to the management of the diagnosis of breast cancer. We wanted to give women the benefit of our own research and experience to help them think beyond their fear when confronted with a possible breast cancer diagnosis. We also wanted to focus on the successful communication and interaction between medical professionals and the woman facing this problem.

Dr. Petrek helps guide us in formulating a list of questions for any woman, regardless of her background or location, to ask of a medical specialist to gain the most recent information on breast cancer treatment. We want to provide all women with the informational tools that will allow her to take control of the process of the diagnosis.

Personally, I knew that I would feel comfortable making decisions only if I thoroughly looked into the breast cancer issue and the available options. I learned that other women wanted the same information but were not sure about how to begin their own personal investigation. The thought of having breast cancer is enough to immobilize even the most confident of women. A sense of being overwhelmed, isolated, and very much out of control faces anyone with the possibility of breast cancer.

I found that many women who have had breast cancer didn't take immediate action when they suspected a problem; they delayed and denied their own good instincts, wasting the precious time that is so necessary in an early diagnosis. This is in large part due to a lack of good information about how to proceed once you find a lump in your breast.

There are many questions, and women aren't sure where to go for the answers. We wonder what the lump means and if it is malignant. Then what? With whom should we consult about this? Is our own doctor qualified to deal with it? Who is? Should we get another opinion? Would a larger hospital be better for us? Where should we look for quality information? How can we deal with this wrenching news? The family? The finances? The fear?

Concrete information is the most important weapon we have to enable us to formulate a plan of action and educated decisions about the process of the disease, the risks involved, and the course of appropriate treatment.

A variety of books and scientific data about breast cancer are available, but I had to learn the hard way that the appropriate information isn't always easy to find when you need it. Sifting through books, periodicals, journals, medical papers, pamphlets, and articles on the subject can be enlightening and also confusing. We cannot possibly expect to know everything about breast cancer, but we can become more informed medical consumers. People who participate in their health care live longer and with a greater sense of well-being.

We have tried in *A Step-by-Step Guide to Dealing With Your Breast Cancer* to approach the subject of the diagnosis logically; to provide truly useful information, arranged and covered in a firm yet sensitive manner; and to direct any woman to ask the difficult questions not only of herself but of the medical professionals with whom she will meet.

Unfortunately, no one definitive process is involved in the diagnosis and treatment of breast cancer. There are, however, certain procedures that most cancer specialists recommend when diagnosing and treating this disease. *A Step-by-Step Guide to Dealing With Your Breast Cancer* is designed to provide direction by informing women in a timely fashion what diagnostic and medical procedures may be required, where to look for the most definitive treatment, how to sort through the process of selecting specialists and hospital facilities, what to ask of medical professionals to determine the latest in surgical options, and what the financial impact will be on their budgets, and ultimately how to make the necessary decisions.

So often, people, and especially women, when confronted with a diagnosis of cancer, feel compelled to follow the course of treatment recommended by the doctor who delivered their original diagnosis. I felt that way and I am sure you might also. Truthfully, it does seem much easier than starting from scratch with another doctor. However, while you may feel comfortable with him or her, you, and those people who are helping you cope, can no longer sensibly perpetuate the myth of blind faith in one physician without question. Dr. Petrek, as do most good doctors, suggests that you seek a second opinion consultation with another specialist.

You, as I did, will be required to gather crucial information in a relatively short period of time on a subject about which you know very little. You need to understand your specific breast cancer and the ways in which it can be treated so that you can evaluate the quality of your medical diagnosis and care. Specific and very useful written information is available to increase your knowledge, but successful communication with the medical professionals with whom you consult is the best method for acquiring the most up-to-date information. *A Step-by-Step Guide to Dealing With Your Breast Cancer* will provide you with a database of resources, indicate which sources will be most useful, and suggest questions that will be invaluable as you meet with the specialists to learn about your breast cancer.

Most women mistakenly think that their doctors will make the important treatment decisions. Realistically, however, the physician will only make a recommendation, and you must make the final decision. If you think that sounds isolated, it is. The diagnosis of breast cancer goes far beyond the breast. It touches us, our loved ones and families, to our emotional core, and such strong emotions cloud our judgment. We face some very difficult choices that will alter our lives, and we are the only ones who can evaluate the physical and emotional effects of our choices and the impact of our decisions.

My experience described in *A Step-by-Step Guide to Dealing With Your Breast Cancer,* along with Dr. Petrek's experience in treating many patients, can help any woman create a strategy that will take her from the first suspicion through treatment. She can then make serious choices and decisions with the conviction that they are right for her.

When I began my personal investigation into this disease, "cancer" literally became my career. I have helped guide many women through the process of diagnosis that I used myself. I have continuously refined and expanded on the process as a result of speaking with women who have also had breast cancer.

Dr. Petrek tries to improve and strengthen her communication and treatment techniques with all her patients. She strives to explain and simplify the diagnostic process to women when organizing their care.

The security of having this plan of action will be especially helpful when you are feeling afraid, anxious, pressured, depressed, and angry that you need to be doing this at all. You will learn how to gather support from your family and from all the people dedicated to curing your breast cancer. You will know what to ask in order to receive direction and positive reinforcement from "your" health care professionals. You will learn that you can manage your emotions and gain strength to help you cope with the disease and prevent you from becoming a victim of it.

A friend once said that I learned courage from having breast cancer. I never thought of myself as courageous, but I think that of every woman who has had to battle breast cancer.

Because of my personal experience and Dr. Petrek's dedication, we can help you organize the diagnosis processes, sort through and understand the procedures that you will be likely to encounter, and help you in your search for the best in health care. You must have the important information at hand to make the difficult choices should you be faced with the possibility of a breast cancer diagnosis.

This book is not a substitute for sound medical advice. It will enable you to work together with your doctor to extract the best possible medical information. Remember, information and communication are the key elements to achieving a healthy return on your life.

Rebecca Robinson
June, 1994

PART ONE

Suspicion

CHAPTER 1

Self-Discovery

Rebecca: Breast cancer. I know about breast cancer. Every week another newspaper, magazine, or newscast has an article or story on yet another well-known person who has developed breast cancer. As women, we naturally discuss among ourselves the numbers of women, many of them our friends, who have had "it." We regularly hear of new information on the disease, its causes, and treatment. I read, I am well informed, I know American Cancer Society statistics state that one in eight women will develop breast cancer at some time during their life. I don't fall into any category that would indicate that I am a candidate for getting breast cancer.

That is what I smugly thought to myself. After all, I take care of myself! I eat properly, I exercise regularly, I don't have any gross overindulgences, I have annual checkups with my gynecologist, I periodically examine my breasts for changes, and I have regular mammograms. I just won't be one of those one in eight American women who will get this disease. Not me!

Have you found yourself saying the same thing?

Most women have very little concrete information about breast cancer and a wealth of misinformation about the disease. I remember a discussion I had with Pat, a very successful woman on the New York arts scene. We were discussing breast cancer, and she told me that she couldn't get it because her breasts were too small. Another woman, Marge, said that she stopped seeing a friend who developed breast cancer because

3

she feared she would get it too. These are just two of the many misconceptions that hinder early diagnosis.

What I failed to realize was that all women are at significant risk. Then I found a small lump in my breast. It was during one of my irregular breast self-examinations, usually performed in bed with the lights out...when my husband was asleep. Isn't it strange how embarrassed and awkward and frightened we feel touching our breasts. We are ashamed to touch them; self-conscious of our body's natural response at our touch and afraid of what we might find if we examine them closely. As women, we spend a great deal of time and money on their rise and support but we ignore them as a part of the body needing medical observation, care, and attention.

Like most women, I am concerned about my appearance, knowing full well the importance of image, both personally and professionally. We, by nature, are proud and protective of our bodies. As we enter puberty and change from girls to women we begin a lifelong consciousness of our breasts. Perhaps this is why we may choose to ignore any troubling suspicions. I have read many books and case histories and there doesn't seem to be any particular pattern to why women do or do not have mammograms on guidelines established by the American Cancer Society.

A friend of mine, Sarah, an investment banker in New York, has a family history of breast cancer. Her mother died from it, and her sister had it a few years ago. When I asked her when she last had a mammogram, she told me three years ago. She is over fifty and has very large breasts. She tells me she just doesn't have the time but she also says she is frightened at what it might reveal.

Dr. Petrek: You know, informal studies have proven that most women, even those at high risk, don't perform breast self-examination with any regularity. We try to ignore our breasts, as if any problem that arises will take care of itself. As we practice our daily bathing rituals we cannot help but notice a new thick area or actual lump, changes in a nipple, either a sore, flaking, or discharge, or a recent inversion where there was none. There could also be dimpling of the skin or a rash on the breast. We might also notice swelling under the arm or around the collarbone. These are some of the external signs that make us suspicious, yet we often choose to ignore them.

Rebecca: You are right. Once a year I work the phone bank at the American Cancer Society for their Breast Cancer Awareness Week. I can't tell you how many women call describing similar problems but are not aware that they could be symptomatic of breast cancer. I wasn't alarmed about my lump because I have lumpy breasts, and these lumps have always shifted and disappeared by the same time in my next monthly cycle. That was my normal pattern.

Dr. Petrek: A large percentage of women will develop lumpy breasts but lumpy breasts do not mean increased risk for breast cancer. Your breasts, like those of most women, are responsive to the physiological events going on within your body. These irregular lumps can and do change in size and number from one menstrual period to the next. Your breasts usually will become very round, swollen, and tender to the touch due to the increase in hormone production that occurred just before your period. It is those hormones that produced this cyclical swelling. Painful, lumpy breasts are due to benign fibrous changes or fluid-filled cysts and are loosely called fibrocystic changes.

Rebecca: I remember being examined by a woman gynecologist many years ago, and I asked her how I would know the difference between the routine lumps and the suspicious lumps. She explained it to me this way: Suppose you are walking alone in your neighborhood, a walk you have taken hundreds of times before, and one day during your walk you sense something amiss, an inexplicable change that makes you suspect there might be a problem. She told me to be alert; some lumps are normal, but one that is new and is around after the next menstrual period should be checked. I had assumed that my lump was to be no different than the others. Still, I was a little uneasy and during the next few weeks I kept checking to see if it had disappeared. Not a day passed that I didn't have thoughts about the possible significance of this lump about the size of a lima bean.

It was March, however, and we were planning a family reunion out West for some serious skiing. With the mechanics of coordinating a vacation as well as my other obligations, I really didn't have the time to let the psychological effects of living with this knowledge get me down. Besides, it would be another month before I could sensibly take any action. I rationalized that it had been one year since my last mammogram, and I had received a thorough examination by my gynecologist just two months ago. I welcomed the opportunity to spend two weeks in the Rockies to clear my mind and exercise my body with those people most dear to me.

For the duration of my holiday I was never completely free of the worry about the lump. In fact, I secretly examined my breasts in the morning shower and late in the evening in bed. I was angry at myself because I had not been more diligent about breast self-examination (BSE). If this lump were serious, perhaps I could have uncovered it earlier.

I knew that BSE should be performed by the menstruating woman every month in the first week after the end of her period and at the same time each month if she no longer menstruates. I did perform BSE, but at infrequent intervals; and, I was not sure now that I knew my breasts as intimately as I should. The idea is to become so familiar with your breasts that you will be able to detect the slightest change from what is normal for you. I just wasn't sure.

The vacation was a success, but on the 4-hour flight home I thought about what I should do about the lump. I realized that I had always taken my good health for granted. Aside from routine gynecological and physical exams and pregnancy, I had very little contact with physicians. I had been in the hospital only twice in my life; once for an emergency appendectomy and once for childbirth. I was ashamed at my lack of knowledge about medicine, doctors, and hospitals. Where should I begin? Who should I see first?

Then I thought about breast cancer. What if this lump was in fact cancer. What would I do?

First, I thought about having a mastectomy and losing the breast. My breasts were never my most attractive feature but they were mine—both of them—and important to me.

Then, I thought that if the lump was malignant I was surely going to die. Perhaps not now or not soon, but eventually the cancer would get me. What did I know about cancer? Not much. What did I know about breast cancer? Not much. Once again I was ashamed at my lack of knowledge.

Next my mind turned to breast self-examination. I knew how to perform BSE and yet I was not confident how long this lump had been around. I had only recently discovered it, and I had been examined by a professional just two months before, and it had not been detected at that time. I tried to remember the pictures in the pamphlets that I had seen in the doctor's office. I tried to re-create in my mind the proper method of examining myself.

Dr. Petrek Explains Breast Self-Examination

Dr. Petrek: The American Cancer Society suggests that BSE should be done once every month at the same time each month by women twenty years of age and older. If you menstruate, the best time to examine your breasts would be seven days after your period begins. The hormone cycle changes, and a wait of seven days will reflect that change when the breasts are less painful and smoother. If you no longer have your period, you should select a day, perhaps the first day of the month, and examine your breasts on that day each month.

BSE is performed in three steps: a visual examination; a manual examination sitting or standing; and a manual examination lying down. First, you stand in front of a mirror and look at your breasts. Inspect the shape of them for dimpling, flattening, puckering, or very rarely, scaling, or a rash, on the skin that may mean trouble. Observe the nipple. Is there a recent inversion or irregularity or a spontaneous discharge? As you watch your breasts assume different positions. Raise your hands and arms above your head, then clasp your hands behind your head and push your head forward. Then, place your hands on your hips and attempt to push your hips inward on both sides. You should be aware of how your breasts look and what is normal for you.

You can perform the manual examination sitting, standing or while you are in the shower. With one arm raised, use the first three fingers to firmly explore your breast under the raised arm in either a circular fashion or a vertical movement beginning at the outer edge near the armpit. Gradually palpate the breast in as many circles or vertical lines as necessary ending with the nipple.

Give attention to the pressure you exert on the breast during your examination. You can usually feel the ribs through the breast tissue. You can be more certain of an accurate breast exam since the breast tissue is being flattened out enough to feel the ribs underneath.

Also, probe the area between the breast and the armpit and then the armpit itself. There is breast tissue under your arm as well as lymph nodes and you are looking for any suspicious lump. Repeat the entire examination on the other breast.

Finally, lie down on your back with your arm over your head so that your breast is flat. Use the same circular rotation or vertical motion and pressure on both breasts as performed in the prior manual examination. Repeat the examination on the other breast. Take the time that you need to perform BSE completely and thoroughly. Have you done this correctly? Have you been this thorough?

If performed correctly, you are a better breast examiner for the individual nature of your breasts than the best physician breast specialist who has been able to examine your breasts only once. You can be an expert in recognizing your own individual anatomy, which varies so greatly from person to person.

Taking Positive Action

Rebecca: I looked over at my husband and son and realized that I had so much to lose. The vacation had been all that I had wanted—a combination of family, sun, steep terrain, and deep powder. However, this lump had me concerned. I knew that this was a critical time. It would have been so easy to ignore the lump. I could, quite naturally, deny, rationalize, and postpone taking any action. I can tell you that the level of anxiety is very high at this time. Even so, I could not in good conscience fail to take action out of fear of what I would discover.

When we arrived home I had decided that the first person

I should call was my gynecologist. This made sense to me for two reasons: First, because I had been his patient for over fifteen years and I trusted him. Second, since the breast is such a uniquely feminine part of the body a gynecologist would have examined many breasts and seen many lumps in the course of his practice. He would have greater knowledge about breasts and their problems. What follows is an account of the action that I took in dealing with my breast lump and a plan for managing the breast cancer diagnosis.

CHAPTER 2

....

Strategic Lifeline

Rebecca: The Strategic Lifeline is a systematic plan that we have developed from our own experiences. Mine in dealing with my breast cancer diagnosis and Dr. Petrek's as a result of years of patient interaction. Through personal trial and error and the experiences of other women, we developed a course of action beginning from the first moment you discover a suspicious breast lump through those procedures and experiences often associated with the breast cancer diagnosis.

When I first suspected that I might have breast cancer I began to search for information that would help me decide what I should do. At that time two things were immediate and enormously helpful. The first was Suzanne, my husband's sister-in-law, who had for the last ten years been in treatment for breast cancer. She had seen the disease firsthand, from the good, to the bad, to the ugly. She had personally dealt with almost all aspects of breast cancer in an effort to control and cure her disease. I knew I could call on her at any time with my questions, also knowing that if she couldn't answer them she could suggest someone who might help me.

The second thing, and also invaluable, was a file that I had kept with a few articles on breast cancer. I am somewhat of an informational pack rat; I maintain clip files on a variety of subjects that might be useful to me either now or at a later date. Why a file on breast cancer? I'll never know, but at least it gave me enough information to begin an investigation.

The Strategic Lifeline should serve as a guide, much in the

way Suzanne and my files were to me. It should help you to understand the process of the breast cancer diagnosis and help you develop a plan of your own that will be helpful during the period of investigating your own options and through to your ultimate treatment.

Dr. Petrek: There are certain standard procedures and tests that can be performed or suggested to confirm a potential diagnosis of the disease. Not all of the tests or procedures on the Lifeline will be ordered by your doctor, as individual cases vary. Each medical specialist has his or her preferred methods for diagnosing and treating breast cancer. Your responsibility is to be aware of what the processes and procedures are, what options are available, and what you will need to know that will allow you to work with the specialist for the best in up-to-date information and quality health care.

Rebecca: The Lifeline is divided into three sections arranged in the order that they will actually take place in the disease process: Confirmation, Investigation, and Treatment. Each section will outline and summarize the process and procedures you may need to successfully diagnose and treat your breast cancer. Each action item on the Lifeline will be covered in greater detail in subsequent chapters throughout the book. Checklists at the end of each chapter will assist you in preparing your own questions for your doctors. Let us now follow the Lifeline so that you will have an overview of what you can expect to happen when you are confronted with a suspicious breast lump.

Confirmation

The First Step—Your Doctor

Let us suppose that you have what you think is a suspicious thickening or a lump in your breast. The first person you would probably want to see is the gynecologist who has been examining your breasts as part of your annual checkups. If you do not have a gynecologist but you do see an internist or a family doctor then call him or her for an appointment.

Like most doctors he schedules patients four to six weeks in advance, but don't let that deter you. Tell the receptionist that you have a suspicious breast lump and that you would like an immediate appointment. If you are able to speak to the doctor, he may at that time refer you to another doctor or specialist more experienced in dealing with breast lumps.

If you do not have a doctor you can call your local chapter of the American Cancer Society for the name of a hospital, medical clinic, or doctor who can see you. Many organizations in this country can help you get good medical care, even if you have no insurance or little money. (Refer to the Database in Part Five for a listing of agencies in your state that can help.)

The doctor you see will perform another breast examination to evaluate the lump. You want medical confirmation that there is in fact a lump, and you would like the doctor's judgment on how you should proceed. He cannot tell you if the lump is malignant. That can only be determined by a biopsy and accurate pathology report.

Diagnostic Tests

Dr. Petrek: Your doctor should arrange for you to have a mammogram if you have not had one within the past six months. Even if you did have one done recently he may still want you to have another. Any mammogram should be done on a machine that is used only for mammograms in a hospital, or in an outpatient radiologist's office, or at a clinic that performs mammograms. You may also have an ultrasound examination at the same time. (Refer to chapter 4 on diagnostic procedures for information about the mammogram and other tests and how to check on the reputation of the facility.) With the results of your mammogram the radiologist should contact your doctor, and they both will help you decide what to do next.

If your mammogram is negative or shows nothing suspicious, and your doctor is convinced that a suspicious lump exists, he or she will want to have the lump tested and/or removed for a complete biopsy. If there is uncertainty about the lump, a delay after another menstrual period may be useful to see if the "lump" disappears and the biopsied area feels only like normal tissue. By taking this approach the doctor may avoid a biopsy on what could be benign temporary changes in the breast.

Should it be necessary, the doctor and the radiologist should recommend that you see a breast surgeon specialist or a general surgeon who is experienced in breast care to perform the biopsy. Ask specifically for the names of several specialists that you can contact, preferably practicing at different hospitals. (Refer to Part Three Investigation, chapters 8 and 9, to help you prepare and research the specialists and hospitals.)

As you are searching for a breast specialist, you will want to think about how the lump should be surgically handled. You have two choices at this point. The less suspicious lump might be treated as a typical benign lump. The more suspicious lumps should be treated as a possible breast cancer. A large percentage of breast lumps are proven to be benign, but in the event of a malignancy the pathology of the lump becomes critical. Also, if the lump proves to be cancer, a second surgical cut to your breast may be needed to take additional breast tissue.

Rebecca: With regard to my own breast cancer, all the medical professionals that I saw told me that the lump was probably nothing more than a cyst. Well, it wasn't, and the edges (margins) of the lump were not clear after the surgery. The surgical margins still contained cancerous roots, as known by the pathologist's report from the first biopsy. Additional surgery was necessary to remove and analyze more breast tissue. Keep this in mind when you are searching for a breast specialist, as more experience may make your course of treatment quicker and it may be possible to have one procedure on the breast instead of two.

Once you have made a decision on the surgeons you will see, make the appointment as quickly as possible. Once again, explain the urgency of your suspicious lump and you will no doubt be seen quickly.

Medical Tests

Dr. Petrek: The breast surgeon will perform a manual examination in the same manner as your gynecologist. He or she may also perform a needle biopsy, which is a mildly uncomfortable insertion of a needle into the breast lump to remove some cells. (Refer to Part Two, chapter 5, regarding the needle biopsy.)

The results of this needle biopsy can take a few days or a week. Question the surgeon about the lab doing the analysis on the lump. When will the report be expected? Is it a large hospital pathology department or a commercial lab? (Refer to Part Two, chapter 6, for information on Pathology.)

The wait can be agonizing and you want to minimize the stress on yourself. In the meantime, the specialist may want to schedule an appointment to perform a surgical biopsy. This is done in an outpatient clinic or surgery department of a hospital.

Rebecca: I discovered that the hospital surgical floor is booked just like any other office or facility. It is important to schedule this appointment as soon as possible and hope that the needle biopsy is fine and you won't need it!

Dr. Petrek, I've heard that many hospitals are using a new procedure called a stereotactic automated large-core biopsy, or simply, a core biopsy. Is this simple procedure as accurate as a surgical biopsy?

Dr. Petrek: Let me explain the difference. Most cancer centers and many other hospitals as well as outpatient areas are currently using stereotactic biopsy. However, this procedure is used almost exclusively on abnormalities seen on a mammogram that are not felt upon manual examination.

There are advantages to using the stereotactic biopsy. First, there is no surgical scar from an incision; second, only local anesthesia is needed; and third, the procedure is done on an outpatient basis and is therefore less expensive.

A more common approach is the surgical biopsy. This is a procedure performed under local anesthesia only or monitored sedation, and general anesthesia is only rarely required. If the lump is large enough, it can be tested in the hospital lab immediately. The test is called a frozen section analysis, and you should know the results before you leave the hospital that day. Your surgeon can tell you whether it is malignant or not. If the lump is small, a frozen section analysis would be difficult to do, and the lump would be sent to pathology in its entirety for analysis. A complete written pathological report on your lump will be made and sent to your doctor upon completion of other laboratory tests.

Rebecca: It can take from several days to over a week to receive this report. The wait can be stressful, but I realize the importance of the pathology report in breast cancer treatment. A woman should ask her doctor what specific tests will be done on her tumor and get the name and telephone number of the laboratory examining the lump so that she may pick up the slides if needed for a second opoinion. (Refer to Part Two, chapter 6, Pathological Diagnosis, for a list of questions you should ask of your doctor.)

Investigation

Your worst suspicions have been confirmed—you have a malignant tumor in your breast. After the initial shock has worn off and you have had a good cry, you realize that you have a million questions to ask. Of whom? To what end? This is a critical time in your mental well-being. You can give in to the anger, self-pity, fear, and denial, or you can try to force yourself to get a grip on the situation.

I decided to do the latter but not without the strength and encouragement of family and friends. I had to educate myself about breast cancer, and you should too. Specifically, about your breast cancer. You have already identified that you have a problem and you are now going to try to enlist the aid of your family and friends and research the problem to the best of your abilities by reading, writing, and discussing breast cancer. You need accurate information about your options to give yourself the best chance for a cure.

My initial reaction when I learned my lump was indeed cancer was to get it removed quickly. All of it. I had to force myself to slow down and take the time to think about a plan that would really be best for me.

Dr. Petrek: It is unwise and not at all necessary to feel that you must have immediate surgery when your tumor is discovered. Most doctors will recommend that you take a reasonable amount of time, usually two or three weeks between diagnosis and surgery, to secure second opinions, seek additional medical consultations, and have additional tests.

While you do not need to feel forced into making decisions prematurely, you will have to act quickly to schedule the second opinion consultations and other tests within the time frame of one or two weeks. (Refer to Part Three, chapters 8 and 9, to help you in preparing a list of specialists, researching the hospital, and meeting the specialist.)

Rebecca: I think one of the most important reasons for engaging in an all-out investigation is the peace of mind you will have several years from now when you are cured. I have met so many women who have regretted the fact that they did not fully research their diagnosis. They live with concern that their cancer was hurriedly and inappropriately treated and fear that it will return. The more information you have will increase your understanding of breast cancer and it will be easier to make the difficult decisions with clarity and confidence.

Test Results and Reports You Need

One of the first things I did once my cancer was confirmed was to obtain the physical evidence of my examinations. If you do not already have a copy of your mammogram X rays you will have to ask your doctor or radiology laboratory for them, along with any report that the radiologist might have written that describes your X rays and his or her examination of you. A written official report is always required when an X ray is performed, and it might take a few days before the dictation is transcribed to be signed by the doctor. If you have had additional tests, such as ultrasound, obtain copies of the results of those tests for your files. (Refer to Part Two, chapter 4, for explanations of diagnostic procedures.)

You will want several duplicate copies of the written medical evaluations of the tests and if possible, have a second copy of your mammogram X rays as well. This may seem like over-organization but when you are dealing with the many people involved in a cancer diagnosis, you want any and all information at hand. Believe me, the process is complicated enough without the added bother of the business aspects of medicine.

Dr. Petrek: You will remember that at the time of your surgical biopsy a frozen section of your tumor may have been taken, while you were still in surgery or immediately thereafter, to determine whether or not your lump was malignant. The remainder of the lump was sent to a pathologist for more detailed laboratory analysis. The laboratory prepares slices of your tumor and transfixes them on glass slides for microscopic examination. Within a few days of your biopsy, you or your surgeon will be notified that the tissue slides of your tumor and an official report are prepared and ready for you to collect and to take with you for your second opinion consultations.

Rebecca: Right. But this can take up to a week and if they are not ready, you need to keep calling the lab. If possible, pick up the slides yourself. I have heard horror stories of lost or missing tumor slides. When you receive them make certain that you are also given a written report from the pathologist.

Dr. Petrek: There will also be a report that will contain information about the hormone receptor composition of your tumor. This report will be an estrogen receptor assay (ERA) and progesterone receptor assay (PRA) that measures the amounts of estrogen and progesterone receptors contained in your tumor. In the past the estrogen and progesterone receptor tests needed to be performed on fresh tissue. A new technique has been developed to perform this test on fixed or previously prepared tissue, even from tissue prepared years ago.

This is important information for your doctors. The medical oncologist will make follow-up treatment recommendations based on the estrogen and progesterone receptor tests. Sometimes the reports of the biopsy and hormonal assays are ready simultaneously, but not always. You will want to make several copies of this report because any professional with whom you consult will want a copy for his or her files.

The slides are an important factor in seeking second opinions and can often be made in duplicate. In fact, hospitals and labs are required to keep a block of your tumor preserved for several years to be used for additional analysis if needed. The other surgeons that you interview would want to review the slides or have the pathologist at his or her hospital look at them before making a recommendation for your treatment.

Rebecca: You will also be confronted with numerous forms and questions about your own medical history, your family's medical history, and your lifestyle habits from birth for each doctor, hospital, and test. Doctors and many other medical professionals, especially those associated with cancer centers and academic health centers, often keep what appear to be unrelated details of their patients. This information can be useful in the research of breast cancer and eventually bring about improvements in the diagnosis and treatment of the disease.

I learned that it helps to have a chronological outline of important medical milestones in your life prepared in advance. This saves in time and frustration at having to re-create one for each doctor. (Refer to Part Two, chapter 7, for a sample outline of the Cancer Worksheet.)

In review, you will want to have with you when you seek second opinions or see other doctors:

1. The mammogram X ray, preferably in duplicate
2. Copies of the written report that describes your mammogram
3. Copies of printouts and evaluations of other tests and/or scans that you have had
4. The tissue slides of your tumor, preferably in duplicate
5. Copies of the complete written report from the pathologist
6. An outline of your medical history

Second Opinion Specialists

At this time, since it has been determined that you have breast cancer, you probably will have met with the surgeon who performed your biopsy either once or twice. The doctor, if he or she is a breast specialist, will have reviewed your slides and has probably made recommendations to you regarding what type of surgery and follow-up treatment you need. He or she undoubtedly would like you to schedule operating room time as soon as possible. The doctor should encourage you to seek a second or third opinion but may not provide you with the names of other surgeons for you to see.

Providing the names of other doctors is sometimes considered equal to recommending them. For example, in some legal cases not only the doctor who made the mistake was sued, but also the doctor who recommended the mistaken doctor to the patient. This is the business of breast cancer. It is important that you try to seek out the top breast cancer specialists in your area for your second and third opinion consultations. How do you find them? (Refer to Part Three, chapter 8, for a complete guide to finding specialists.)

The gynecologist you originally saw when the lump was discovered should give you some names for referral. Also, you should advise your family physician about what is going on, since he or she is familiar with your medical history. Both doctors should be able to recommend one or two specialists. Your insurance company or HMO may also have a list of specialists to recommend, and they may require you to use one of their doctors for both your second opinion and for your treatment.

I found it helpful to ask at work and have my husband ask around at his office also. You will be surprised at the information you can get from business contacts. You can also call the largest hospital in your area to obtain a list of breast specialists.

Unfortunately, there is no board certification for breast surgeon specialists nor is there any certification for cancer surgeon specialists. Breast specialists are those who have board certification in general surgery, expertise in cancer surgery, and then have specialized in treatment of the breasts. In smaller cities a breast specialist might also treat cancer of other areas.

If you do not have any contacts or friends with names of doctors, regional and national organizations can help you. (Refer to Part Five, the Database, for the names and numbers to call.) Do not overlook your regional unit of the American Cancer Society. It can provide you with the names of leading doctors and Regional Cancer Centers in your area.

The United States currently has twenty-five Comprehensive Cancer Centers recognized by the National Cancer Institute that are strategically located and listed in the Database. Find the center nearest you and call for the names of their breast cancer specialists. The National Cancer Institute in Bethesda, Maryland (800-4-CANCER), publishes communications materials to assist patients in finding the names and addresses of qualified specialists, other cancer centers, and breast cancer programs in their area.

In your search for a specialist you will find that one or two doctors in your area seem to handle the majority of breast cancer cases. Consider the sources of the recommendations carefully. Some doctors have many breast cancer patients because so many women seem to be getting breast cancer. They have had to treat women out of necessity. The theory of supply and demand has generated numbers of patients, but many of these doctors are not specialists. The doctors you should want to call for a consultation or second opinion are the specialists. I know that it can be inconvenient to see them, especially if there is travel involved, but you will not regret having made the effort. Because you have your mammogram X rays, tissue slides, and pathologist report, you should be able to schedule an appointment within a few days. Breast surgeons recognize the immediacy of your problem and will make every effort to accommodate you.

What to Ask

Dr. Petrek: Before you have your consultations, you will want to organize the information that you have accumulated and prepare a list of questions to ask the doctor. You should want to know why one surgical procedure is recommended over another; how many operations of that type the doctor performed; what additional tests or scans he or she requires; what is planned for follow-up care; if additional treatment is indicated; and, of course, how much it will cost.

When you are preparing your list of questions it is helpful to divide them between the secretary, the nurse, and the surgeon. For example, at large hospitals the secretary usually handles the billing and will know exactly what items cost and how to organize in dealing with your insurance company or HMO. The nurse will be valuable to discuss the aftercare of the surgical incision and other specific details of the surgery. The nurse can connect you with a social worker regarding your hospital stay or to discuss the psychological aspects of breast cancer. Each woman will have questions that relate to her own personal medical case history. (Refer to Part Three, chapter 8, for guidance in formulating a list of questions for the specialist.)

Rebecca: The exchange of information can be very detailed and lengthy. Bring your husband or a friend with you who can take notes. And, if the doctor allows it, I recommend that you bring a microcassette tape recorder. I found this invaluable bcause I could review the dialogue under less stressful circumstances.

Truthfully, I just couldn't digest everything in that one meeting. Also, I was upset and frightened at what the doctor was saying and not thinking clearly. On the one hand, I didn't want to be on the receiving end of this consultation, but then again I didn't want to miss any information either.

Treatment

Dr. Petrek: My research on recent developments in breast cancer treatment and the personal case histories of the women that I see indicate that breast cancer is most successfully treated by multidisciplinary specialists or several doctors that work together on your case. I realize that successful treatment is purely subjective and solely dependent on cure and quality of life.

Rebecca: Of the women I interviewed, those who were most confident that they received the best treatment had a team of doctors watching over them and had taken advantage of the services offered at a multidisciplinary center. Personally, at my hospital, the surgeon was in communication with the medical oncologist and the radiation oncologist about my treatment. The medical oncologist and radiation oncologist were debating, each with my cure in mind, the timing of my radiation treatment and my chemotherapy. The psychiatric social worker, the group therapy sessions, and the physical therapist all contributed to my quick and complete recovery.

Dr. Petrek: At many large hospitals and cancer centers you may meet several staff specialists in one visit to discuss possible treatments. With this team approach you can meet with a breast surgeon, a plastic surgeon (if you choose immediate or subsequent breast reconstruction after mastectomy), and a radiation oncologist. At a different appointment after surgery you can meet with a medical oncologist.

Since each specialist has access to your medical profile, they will outline a treatment plan that is right for you. The multidisciplinary second opinion approach to breast cancer treatment serves two purposes for you. First, you can discuss every aspect of what you can expect in the form of treatment options from several sources. And second, you are assured that several specialists are involved in your treatment and watching your progress. There is no substitute for that peace of mind and confidence from knowing that several professionals are engaged in the details of your treatment and can check and cross-check on one another.

Your Decision

Rebecca: You are now at the point where you should make treatment decisions based on your consultations with medical specialists and the information you have accumulated. The doctors will not make the decision on what type of treatment you will need. They will only offer their recommendations on what, in their opinion, is the best form of treatment for your case. Ultimately, you are responsible for deciding upon the course of treatment you want based on how far your cancer has progressed, the type of breast surgery recommended to you, how much follow-up therapy you might need, and how you feel about your breast cancer in relationship to your general health.

I found this absolutely frightening. Here we were, my husband and I, trying to decide how I would be treated for cancer. You will be weighing lifelong views about your body image against your preconceived ideas about cancer. Ultimately, however, no one can evaluate how you will feel about the decision except yourself. Fortunately, you should have researched the subject, interviewed your doctors, and can approach the decision-making process with confidence. (Refer to chapter 15 for help with making the decision.) The confidence factor may not come now because you still have the surgery and subsequent follow-up to go through. It will come, though.

Dr. Petrek: Selecting the specialist to follow through on your treatment choice is a highly personal decision. Once you have chosen the specialist that you want to perform your surgery, you will want to schedule the surgery as soon as possible. Keep in mind that operating room schedules and surgical schedules are often full, and it may take some time to find a mutually acceptable date. Your doctor may also want you to have additional tests such as a bone scan or liver scan. These tests can determine if your breast cancer has metastasized or spread beyond the breast to other sites in your body. Both tests are routine and not uncomfortable but will take time to schedule. The hospital will also require that you have a blood workup, electrocardiogram, and chest X ray taken prior to admission.

Organize Yourself

Rebecca: In the meantime, there will be endless forms that need your attention. Surgical consent forms and hospital admission papers have to be filled out. Your insurance company will expect to be notified of your anticipated surgery. By now you will have noticed that no matter where you go or whom you see in connection with your breast cancer, all want certain information from you. I wish someone had advised me of this earlier in my diagnosis. It would have saved me valuable time.

Make life easy on yourself, and carry a folder or briefcase with your insurance card, copies of blank insurance claim forms, written reports, your master calendar, drivers license or proof of identification, checks, and credit cards. Yes, hospitals and some specialists do take credit cards. You can also save considerable time if your insurance claim forms are filled out in advance so that you can leave them when you have your tests or medical visits.

Prepare files for those bills you have already paid and for which you will need insurance reimbursement and for those bills which are to be paid directly by the insurance company. Keep a detailed list of expenses for tax purposes. You will be astounded at the costs connected with breast cancer treatment and the paperwork that it generates. I found that if I didn't keep up with the bills and insurances I not only lost money, but I couldn't prove payment when the hospital made an error. (Refer to chapter 13 on Managing the Finances.)

We hope you have followed the Lifeline using it as a guide to the process of managing your diagnosis and to choosing a course of treatment for yourself and your breast cancer. Once you have completed all the research, you should feel confident with the information you have accumulated about your breast cancer. During my own personal investigation I made many mistakes and I have tried to point out some of those problems that can invariably come with a breast cancer diagnosis. Hopefully, this knowledge, along with active participation in the cancer diagnostic process, will give you the strength to proceed with the surgery you need and the peace of mind that you have helped determine the course of your own life.

STRATEGIC LIFELINE Six Weeks to Treatment	ACTION
Week 1	
Suspicion: discovery of breast lump	Breast self-examination or mammography
Week 2	
Confirmation: medical support for your suspicion	Meet physician, gynecologist, internist, for: Examination Arrange for mammography Have ultrasound or other tests Obtain referral to breast specialist
Prepare:	Copies of mammography Copies of ultrasound Medical History Contact HMO or insurer Schedule breast specialist

Week 3 Appointment with breast specialist	Examines your breast Performs needle biopsy Schedules additional biopsy Receives results of pathology
Prepare:	Receive pathology slides Photocopy pathology reports
Week 4 Investigation: do your own research	Seek out hospitals and specialists

Prepare:	Schedule second opinion
	   consultations, include one
	   multidiscipline meeting
	Formulate a list of questions for
	   the specialists including type
	   of surgery, treatment options
	   and follow-up

Week 5
Decisions: evaluate the options
	Make treatment decisions
	Schedule surgery
	Have additional tests if necessary
	Organize job and personal
	   calendar
	Prepare files for costs and
	   insurances, forms and bills

Week 6
Prehospitalization
	Have required tests and
	   procedures; blood workup,
	   X-rays, EKG, preadmission
	   paperwork

PART TWO

Confirmation

CHAPTER 3

Medical Diagnosis

Rebecca: The Strategic Lifeline has provided an overview of the process that could take place when a woman is confronted with a suspicious lump in her breast. We now need to be more specific about what the medical diagnosis entails and what should be done within reasonable and safe limits to proceed with a medical diagnosis.

Dr. Petrek: By the time you or your doctor have discovered what is diagnosed as a cancer, the malignant cells which cause a lump have probably been growing for some time. If the lump is large, the malignant cells have probably been there for several years. Breast cancer cells can reproduce themselves in as little as six weeks or as long as six months. In general, younger women tend to have more rapidly growing tumors than older women. Today, approximately one quarter of the women diagnosed with breast cancer are premenopausal or under fifty years old.

Rebecca: I remember that when I was in the hospital following my breast surgery, my mother, then in her late sixties, was shocked at the age of the women on my floor with breast cancer. Well over half of us were in our forties, many with small children. Even if you are young, a small lump can be serious. In reading reports issued by the National Cancer Institute, it has been shown that even a small lump, if strategically located, can send microscopic cancer cells to other parts of the body. And, those cancer cells don't always travel through the lymph nodes but can directly enter the bloodstream and travel to other organs.

Dr. Petrek: Most women have fibrocystic changes in their breasts and often breast lumps can change in size or hardness from one month to the next. A suspicious lump is different from prior lumps you might have felt. Breast cysts may become enlarged prior to the onset of a menstrual period and may be smaller between periods. This temporary change in size may vary quite a lot. A delay until after another menstrual period may be useful to see if the lump disappears and the area feels like normal tissue.

A lump that remains the same size from one menstrual period to the next should make you suspicious. A cancerous lump tends to feel as if it is covered in velvet and sticks in the tissue and cannot be moved around easily. A benign lump tends to be slippery and is not exactly round but irregular in shape. Clearly, these signs indicate that this lump should be examined by a physician. There are always exceptions, so that any lump causing any question to any woman should be examined by a physician.

Rebecca: Yes, but very often women are not certain when they detect a lump whether it could be serious or not. Even a woman who performs breast self-examination regularly cannot be entirely sure. Only a thorough examination by a physician can provide confirmation that a suspicious lump exists. A lump that is discovered as the result of routine mammography can sometimes eliminate the guesswork associated with the manual discovery of lumps. Detection by mammography may reveal radiologic characteristics indicating that the lump is most likely a cancer.

For most women the obvious person to contact would be their gynecologist or family physician. He or she is a doctor who is familiar to us and someone in whom we trust. We have been to the office several times, it is familiar to us, and it should be an emotionally easier call to make.

Don't call just to make an appointment with your doctor, however, explain to the nurse or receptionist that you have a suspicious breast lump and you would like to have it examined by the doctor. More than likely, the office will fit you in within a day or two. A delay of several days is fine. Just don't postpone taking any action for much longer. You will feel a great sense of relief from just having made the telephone call to schedule the appointment.

In the interim, try to continue with your daily routine if that will keep you from obsessing over the lump. Some women take comfort in performing routine tasks while others may want an activity that will completely distract them. Do whatever you must to help you remain calm. This is not the time to engage in "what ifs" or imagining the worst. Try not to worry. You can be optimistic; more than 85 percent of biopsied breast lumps are not cancer.

Dr. Petrek: The physical examination that the doctor performs will be similar to those you have always had with him or her. The doctor will have your file with notes from prior examinations and will ask you about your family history, symptoms and suspicions. During this examination the doctor will ask you to sit, raise your arms above your head, then to your side, and finally ask you to place your hands on your hips. The doctor is looking for any obvious visible physical changes.

The doctor will palpate the lymph node areas in your neck, particularly the base of the neck. Normal lymph nodes are small and soft and cannot usually be detected by routine palpation. Firm and enlarged lymph nodes indicate that a problem might exist. The doctor will also examine your armpit or axilla to determine if the lymph nodes there are firm or enlarged. The doctor will then ask you to lie down and he will palpate your breasts. A gynecologist will probably feel your abdomen and pelvis, checking for abnormalities in general.

The experience of your physician is important in evaluating the lump. He has confirmed the presence of a lump and will probably recommend that you have a mammogram in order to obtain more information. Remember, all lumps are suspect until cancer has been ruled out.

Rebecca: I am always bothered when women tell me, and there are many more than I am comfortable with, that they have a lump and the doctor is watching it for the next four or five months. Some women with chronic fibrocystic changes routinely see their gynecologist about breast lumps to watch for any peculiar changes in size or dimension. A friend of mine in New York, an elegant woman in her fifties, has many lumps in both breasts. She and her doctor have made charts on both breasts indicating where the lumps are positioned. At each checkup the charts are reviewed and revised accordingly.

As patients, we tend to think of our doctors as having all the answers, especially the answers we want to hear. This is not always so, and a doctor should refer you to a breast specialist for another opinion, even if the mammogram is normal, because mammograms are not completely accurate depending upon many individual factors. They do not always reveal on film some lumps that are detected by either self-examination or manual examination performed by a physician. This is called a false-negative mammogram. Conversely, a false-positive mammogram will indicate the presence of a tumor where there is none. Across all age groups the rate of mammography not detecting a cancer which is present is 15 percent. However, the percentage would be higher in young women and lower in postmenopausal women. The predominant attitude is that breast lumps which persist through a menstrual period should be removed and their composition should be tested.

I remember when the doctor verified my lump. At first I felt relieved that my mind and my touch were not playing tricks with each other. But then, the anxious feeling about the lump was replaced by more concrete apprehension. I made a list of things that I wanted the doctor to know, such as when and how I first made the discovery, when I had my last checkup, when I had my last period, and other personal concerns. I also listed questions that I needed answered.

You can and should ask your doctor for his judgment on what this lump means and what is likely to happen next. You want to know what his experience has been with breast lumps like yours. Hopefully, you feel comfortable communicating your questions and fears to him or her. After all, this is your doctor, and he or she is genuinely interested in your welfare.

After your physician has examined you and answered your questions he will more than likely want you to have a mammogram. Have him give you the names of two facilities that perform mammography, and preferably other diagnostic tests as well. In my case, my breast cancer did not appear on the mammogram, and an ultrasound test was recommended to measure the size and density of my lump. The differences between the mammogram and the ultrasound are explained in chapter 4 on Diagnostic Procedures. Both tests were performed at the same facility within minutes of one another. It would have been time-consuming and far more stressful to have to reschedule the ultrasound at another facility at another time.

You can also have the doctor's nurse or receptionist make the appointment for you. That way you will be certain of getting the earliest possible appointment. Ask the doctor to give you the names of breast specialists or surgeons with extensive experience in breast care. And ask the doctor why he recommends those particular surgeons.

You can't believe that all this is happening to you. This is not a pleasant experience! Who should you share this information with? You aren't even sure what you've got. The words "breast cancer" creep into your mind, and you can't seem to block them out. This is every woman's nightmare and you are living it!

CHAPTER CHECKLIST

1. You must make that first telephone call to your doctor; you cannot ignore this lump any longer.
2. Be specific and aggressive about your problem; insist on an appointment within the coming week or as soon as possible.
3. Have your list of questions prepared for your doctor. You will want to know how much experience he has with breast problems; what is his method and procedure in dealing with them; where does he recommend that you go for a mammogram and/or diagnostic tests; who does he recommend as a breast specialist that you can see if you need a biopsy.
4. If a mammogram is indicated, and it often is, have your doctor make the appointment then and there. A mammogram might not be required if the woman is in her twenties, for fear of extra radiation at a young age, or if she has had a good quality mammogram in the last three to six months or

so. Inquire if other tests might be indicated. What are they? Why?

5. Keep the appointment. You know you are afraid of what he will tell you, but you also know that 85 percent of biopsied breast lumps are not cancer.

CHAPTER 4

······································

Diagnostic Procedures

Dr. Petrek: Several diagnostic tests are available today performed by licensed radiologists that can aid in the detection and treatment of breast cancer. They are usually the mammogram and ultra sound for testing the breast. A variety of other tests such as nuclear scans, computerized axial tomography (CAT), and magnetic resonance imaging (MRI) can be performed to determine whether cancer has spread to a distant site in your body, such as the liver or bones. These diagnostic tests will be detailed in the following pages.

These tests should be administered in a facility that has been certified by the American College of Radiology and is under the supervision of a full-time, board-certified radiologist. The Food and Drug Administration and the American College of Radiology have issued specific standards of compliance for mammography facilities before they can receive federal certification, beginning in October 1994. The FDA requires that facilities pass accreditation inspections, have specialized high-quality equipment, require that doctors and technicians have training in the specific test areas, maintain accurate records on the tests that are performed at that facility, and finally be audited yearly.

Rebecca: A woman should not assume that because a facility is familiar to her, in her neighborhood or town, that it is certified. She should call the American College of Radiology (703-648-8900) or the National Cancer Institute's information service at (800-4-CANCER) for the names and addresses of those certified breast-imaging facilities nearest her.

Then she should call those facilities recommended and ask what tests and scans are performed at the site and when the equipment was last inspected by a radiological physicist before making the appointment. Because some sites currently are certified only by individual states and not by the American College of Radiology, and you are looking for a facility that is in compliance with the FDA and the Mammography Safety and Quality Act (MSQA). All facilities must be qualified by October 1994.

The skill of the technician who actually takes your X ray or scan is of great importance. He or she should specialize in the specific tests that you are having and should be certified by the American Registry of Radiologic Technologists. You don't want to have to repeat a test due to an error by the technician. The expertise of the radiologist who will be evaluating the results of your test is also very important. He or she should be certified by the American Board of Radiology and the American College of Radiology. You want someone who is experienced in reading the specific test you are having.

The Mammogram

Dr. Petrek: Mammography is the best and most commonly used test for detecting small breast tumors at an early and therefore more curable stage. Mammography can detect breast cancer approximately two or three years before a lump is felt in manual examination. It can also reveal a suspicious shadow or calcium particles that might possibly develop into cancer in the future in currently healthy women. Mammography also can help the doctor in determining whether a palpable lump is malignant or not. It can also give the exact location of a tumor in a woman who does not have a lump but has symptoms such as dimpling, thickening, or nipple disturbances. In addition it can prove helpful in locating unknown tumors in the opposite breast. The availability of the mammogram in early detection has greatly increased the success in treating breast cancer.

Rebecca: Although the mammogram can save women's lives, a large percentage of women still neglect or are afraid to have this simple X ray test. The American Cancer Society estimates that 70 percent of women do not have regular mammograms according to their guidelines. It is alarming that so many women have never had a mammogram. The rationalizations for neglecting to have one can vary from woman to woman, but fear and cost seem to be the most common reasons. Some fears include the fear of disrobing in front of doctors and technicians, fear of repeated X ray exposure, fear of pain or discomfort as the breasts are compressed, and doubts about the accuracy of the mammogram, what it will or will not reveal. Some women feel that because they have no history of breast cancer they don't need to have a mammogram. And other women just aren't aware of the guidelines recommended for mammography.

The American Cancer Society and other health organizations and medical institutions recommend baseline mammograms for women between the ages of 35 to 39. Women aged 40 to 49 should have a mammogram every 1 or 2 years, even if there are no symptoms. Annual mammography is recommended for women 50 and over. Also, women with the significant risk factors that are reviewed in chapter 7 should discuss with their doctors the timing of their mammogram X rays.

Each May I serve as a volunteer on the telephone bank at the American Cancer Society for their Breast Cancer Awareness Week. Women 35 and over who have never had a mammogram and do not have any current breast problems are urged to call and schedule a low cost ($40) mammogram at a certified site near her home or office. Many of the women who call are well over 35, some in their 50s and 60s, and have never ever had a mammogram. In fact, there are many large screening centers nationwide that do hundreds of mammograms weekly, some that charge as little as $50 for the test.

Also, most states have laws that require insurance or HMO reimbursement for a mammogram. You can call your state Department of Health or the state division of the American Cancer Society listed in the Database, Part Five, for information on costs or breast imaging facilities. Cost should not be a deterrent to receiving a quality mammogram.

For many women the prospect of having a mammogram

can bring on a case of the hives, or an upset stomach, or the shakes. This anxiety is very real and can be a typical reaction for many women. For women, this is the most dreaded diagnostic procedure. Perspiration drips from pores you never knew you had and you engage in "what if..." scenarios.

You not only fear the test procedure but you also fear even more what the test might show. As you look around you at the other women in the waiting room you notice that they all look healthy. All of them, however, are obviously distracted and nervous. The bottom line is that seven out of eight women will not develop breast cancer. So take a deep breath, and be confident that you are taking sensible, intelligent action.

Dr. Petrek: Many women are afraid that a mammogram X ray will increase their chance of getting breast cancer because of repeated exposure to the X ray machine. This is not proven. Because today's X ray film is more sensitive than it used to be, better pictures are produced at smaller radiation doses. Modern low-dose mammography equipment uses less than 1 rad per breast, usually between 0.03 to 0.05 rad. At such low levels, the chances of getting breast cancer from the mammogram are insignificant when compared with the benefit of detecting an early cancer. The World Health Organization Committee on Breast Imaging Technologies in Breast Cancer Control states that the risk of mammography for women over 40 is negligible.

Rebecca: The American College of Radiology and the American Cancer Society guidelines suggest that every woman, even those who have no history of breast cancer in their family or who have no symptoms, have a baseline mammogram between the ages of 35 and 40. This "baseline" mammogram will provide a picture of your normal breasts for later comparison with future mammograms. Incidentally, most facilities by law keep mammograms indefinitely although you may keep your own or have a copy made for your own files.

As we age, more of our breast tissue is replaced by fat and the mammogram is more useful as a diagnostic tool. The breast becomes less dense, making it easier to spot a lump on a mammogram. This is especially important for women over 50. Some controversy exists regarding annual mammograms on younger, lower-risk women. Their breast tissue is more dense, thereby making mammograms more difficult to read. Many women at ages 40 to 50, who are considered to be at high risk for breast cancer, should consult with their doctor about having annual mammograms. I know several young women whose mothers have had breast cancer and they insist on early mammograms. What about the accuracy of mammography?

Dr. Petrek: Mammograms are usually accurate, but they have a 15 percent failure rate of not detecting a cancer that actually exists for women of all ages. In other words, the younger patients who have denser breasts have less accuracy expected and the older patients have more accuracy expected.

Rebecca: I had a false-negative mammogram. It detected nothing that would indicate that I had breast cancer although both my physician and I could feel the lump. While a false-negative or -positive mammogram can happen anywhere, it is wise to do some research on the facility where you will be having the mammogram done. Make certain that you ask whether the facility has up-to-date, well-maintained X ray equipment that is used only for mammography. This is called "dedicated" mammography equipment and should be checked twice a year. You want to avoid excessive radiation exposure on old-fashioned equipment.

For those women living in rural areas, it is definitely worth the trip to a regional or university medical center, which will probably have the latest available machines in your area. I just received notification from a small-town hospital in rural New England that they had recently received certification from the American College of Radiology. I was pleased to hear this news, but I know that they have been doing mammograms for years. It made me wonder about the accuracy of the prior mammography.

If you have doubts about the radiologist or the facility, contact the American College of Radiology, 1891 Preston White Drive, Reston, VA 22091 (703-648-8900), or the American Board of Radiology, Suite 440, 300 Park, Birmingham, MI 48009 (313-645-0600). The Food and Drug Administration has issued specific standards of compliance for mammography facilities before they can receive federal certification.

When you must have your mammogram, either routinely

or as a result of a suspicious lump, there are several things that you can do to make the experience as stress-free as possible. Do not put off making the telephone call, or if you are a patient with a special problem, have your doctor make the appointment for you. A delay will not only increase your anxiety but your risk as well. Schedule the appointment for early in the morning when you will be fresh and alert. You will also save yourself that inevitable wait that seems to occur in medical offices as the day progresses. In a nonemergency situation, try to schedule your mammogram immediately following your menstrual period, not just prior to or during your period, when your breasts may be subject to hormonal swelling and are tender.

There are no special eating or drinking requirements prior to a mammogram. However, it is sometimes suggested that you avoid caffeine for a week before the test. You should remember not to use deodorants or powders on your underarms or breasts on the day of your mammogram as some of their ingredients can be seen on the film and interfere.

Dress comfortably and warmly. You will be asked to undress to the waist and will not want to fumble with snaps and buttons. Also, doctor's offices, clinics, and hospitals seem to be climate-controlled and to my mind are always cold. Wear a cardigan sweater or jacket that can be worn over the smock or gown you are given. Don't wear expensive clothes or jewelry; you will be leaving them in a locker or closet.

Bring reading material with you. You may have a wait before your mammogram, while you are in the room waiting for the technician, and while the film is checked to make certain that the breast images are clear.

The technician will position you for the two types of exposures or views, one view from the top and one from the side for each breast. Four pictures in all. For each X ray image the breast will be pressed between two plates. This procedure is uncomfortable but not painful, and the compression is important to produce a good picture. Additional views may be required depending on the shape and size of the breast. Don't be alarmed if this happens.

In some facilities the mammogram will be read immediately by the radiologist, and you will know the results promptly; and at other facilities the radiologist reports the findings to your physician. If you won't know the results that day, ask when you can call your physician for the results. A good facility or clinic will have your mammogram read by a board-certified radiologist immediately.

If your mammogram is normal, you should receive written notification within a week or ten days. Your doctor should also receive a written report.

If your mammogram is questionable, you may be called to return for additional views to be taken of the breast.

If your mammogram indicates an abnormality, you should be telephoned or notified immediately, or if you had a diagnostic mammogram because of a specific problem, your films should be reviewed immediately and the radiologist should discuss the results and any possible action with you at the time of the test. He or she should notify your doctor in writing of the results of the mammography.

Keep in mind that having a mammogram is no more uncomfortable than other tests or procedures to which we routinely subject ourselves. It should be as routine as a trip to the dentist, gynecologist, or family physician for a checkup. The exam takes about 10–15 minutes, and the cost of a mammogram ranges from $75 to $200.

Ultrasound

Dr. Petrek: The ultrasound or "sonogram" test is another important diagnostic tool that is also performed by a radiologist and is useful in detecting and measuring breast lumps that have been found on physical exams and mammography. It is not generally useful for screening. It is a painless, noninvasive test that does not use X rays but instead uses high-frequency sound waves that can detect and distinguish between fluid cysts and a solid lump. The sound waves, not detectable to the human ear, produce different kinds of echos when they touch various tissue or organs. A computer converts the echos into an image that electronically transforms the information into a picture on a video monitor whose screen is mathematically divided in sections to measure variations.

Ultrasound has been used for years on pregnant women because there is no risk of radiation damage when examining the fetus. Ultrasound provides supporting information when a lump is in question. It is particularly useful in obtaining size and shape measurements or texture and densities of a suspected tumor. Ultrasound is also useful if the mammogram is normal, but a lump exists.

Rebecca: Ultrasound is a painless procedure often used in conjunction with the mammogram. In my case, my tumor did not appear on a mammogram but was clearly apparent on the ultrasound test. As I lay on an examining table in a darkened room a technician applied conductor liquid or jelly to the breast to provide good contact with a device known as a transducer. She then gently and slowly moved the transducer over the breast area containing the questionable lump. The breast image was transposed onto a screen that contained measured markings. The ultrasound takes approximately 15 minutes, and costs range from $75 to $250.

Magnetic Resonance Imaging (MRI)

Dr. Petrek: Magnetic Resonance Imaging or the MRI is a useful piece of equipment for imaging parts of the body, but not usually the breast. It is unique in that it is noninvasive and does not expose the patient to any radiation nor any radioactive material. It provides detailed two-dimensional pictures of body tissues that formerly could be seen only by injecting foreign dyes or performing diagnostic surgery. The MRI can see through bone and produce precise computerized images of blood vessels, fluids, cartilage, muscles, ligaments, and bone marrow. It can also detect cancer in specific tissue as well as benign tumors and can be used to study the body chemistry in the various stages of disease. While the MRI test is rarely used in the breast cancer diagnosis, it can be useful if there is suspicion that there might be cancer elsewhere in the body.

The MRI scanner is a tubelike magnetic coil large enough for a person to slide through. You can lie either fully clothed or in a hospital gown on a nonmagnetic cushioned table that is slid into the MRI machine. The machine is narrow but is open at both ends. The test is not uncomfortable and you do not feel anything, but you will be asked to lie very still in the magnetic field. You will also be listening to noises such as loud popping sounds and normal humming machinelike sounds.

The MRI computer analyzes the electromagnetic signals that your body gives off and processes the information it has accumulated throughout the test. The computer then translates the data into a picture of separate body images on a TV monitor. When the scan is finished the images will be viewed for quality and clarity, and then a radiologist will study the images. The results of the scan will be given to your doctor to aid in your breast cancer diagnosis.

Rebecca: The MRI scans may be performed at a hospital, clinic, or outpatient imaging center. When you arrive at the scanning area the radiologist or his technician will inform you about the procedure for your scan. He or she will ask you for a brief medical history and you can ask the technician about any questions or concerns you might have.

To prepare for your exam you will be asked to remove any metal objects from your body that might respond to the magnetic field such as hairpins or hairpieces, glasses, dentures, jewelry, belts, clothes with metal zippers or snaps, coins, and credit cards with magnetic strips. MRI scans should not be used on people with metal objects implanted in their bodies that might be affected by the magnetic field. Such objects include pacemakers, artificial valves or joints, surgical metal clips, or an intrauterine device. Finally, you may be checked with a metal detector as an extra precaution. The exam takes from 30 to 90 minutes, and the cost of MRI is $600 to $1,500.

Nuclear Scans

Dr. Petrek: Often after a diagnosis of breast cancer has been made a physician will order specific nuclear scans. Nuclear scans are additional diagnostic tests that provide the doctor with detailed computerized pictures of specific body areas. They are useful for the doctor to study to determine whether the cancer has spread to other sites in the body such as the bones and liver. This is important knowledge because a woman whose cancer has spread beyond her breast may not necessarily be cured by having breast surgery. Other forms of treatment might be better for her.

A scan is also a useful diagnostic tool in that it can provide a healthy baseline from which to evaluate any future problems that might develop. Nuclear scans are important because they are reliable, have very little risk, and are painless alternatives to many separate X rays. Scans generally expose a patient to less than 10 percent of the radiation from multiple routine X rays. The scans can determine which areas of the body need follow-up X rays rather than subjecting a patient to a variety of X rays at the outset. The most common scans ordered by doctors in determining a breast cancer diagnosis are made of the bones and liver.

The bone scan is used to check the entire body skeleton for breast cancer. This scan is very sensitive and will reveal an abnormal area in the bones, often many months before it can be detected by standard X ray procedures. The liver scans are used to detect and diagnose whether a breast cancer has spread to the liver. Although the bone scans are very specific, if a scan reveals an abnormality, the X ray can provide more detailed analysis of the problem area. If abnormalities are seen on the liver scan, additional tests may be ordered, such as a liver ultrasound to provide additional clarification.

A Computerized Axial Tomography (CAT) scan is not really a nuclear scan but more a form of X ray. It is included here because this test could also be ordered to provide supporting information on the possibility of cancer in other parts of the body. The CAT scan is a sophisticated diagnostic X ray machine that uses radiation to provide detailed photographs of specific areas of the body.

As you lie on a table, the round tubelike machine takes many cross-section pictures of your body. The pictures are then electronically transferred by a computer to produce very detailed photographs of slices or sections of your organs. The procedure takes less than one hour and costs between $500 and $1,000.

Rebecca: The scans are not painful nor do they pose a risk to your health. It is, however, unnerving to find yourself in an area of the hospital that is named "Nuclear Medicine." Although some scans can be performed in a doctor's office, most nuclear tests are given in hospitals. The largest cancer centers, university hospitals, large clinics, and regional medical centers will have nuclear medicine departments. The equipment used to produce the scans is massive, technologically advanced, and very expensive. Because the equipment is complicated, the scans are administered by a team of nuclear medicine specialists.

To insure your safety, the equipment environment and radioactive materials are strictly monitored. You may be required to sign a consent form. This is a contract that explains the diagnostic or medical procedure that you are about to have. When you sign the consent form you agree to undergo the procedure with the understanding and acceptance of the risks as well as the benefits of that procedure.

The scan procedure is simple and takes about three hours from start to finish. The patient is injected in a vein in the arm with a radioactive compound, sometimes called a radioisotope or radiopharmaceutical. The radioisotope usually used in bone scans is technetium-99m and has a lifespan of several hours. The radiation dose is less than 1 rad. Rad is the abbreviated name for "radiation absorbed dose" and a term of measurement used in any radiation treatment. The radioisotope leaves the body quickly, which keeps the radiation exposure to a minimum. This sounds ominous but in fact is like having a blood test.

You will be asked to wait for one hour or more after injection or until the radioisotope is well into your body and adheres to your bones. You are then brought into a room that looks like "command headquarters" and positioned (fully clothed) on a glass table under a large machine called a gamma camera. The camera very slowly moves above your body producing a picture of your skeleton on a computer monitor. It traces the distribution of the radioisotope in the body and records it on photographic film. It was fascinating to look on the monitor and see my skeleton before me.

The results of the scan are read and interpreted by the nuclear medicine physician, a specialist trained in chemistry and physics with specific expertise in the use of radioactive materials in testing. After the evaluation he will contact your physician to discuss possible treatments for you. Scans take from 2 to 3 hours and cost from $300 to $1,000, and most are covered by insurance or medical plans.

In conclusion, all tests, whether they are mammography, ultrasound, the MRI, CAT, or nuclear scans, are designed to help your doctor produce an accurate diagnosis of your breast cancer and administer the appropriate treatment. The radiologists and technicians are specialists and are ready and willing to answer any of your questions and relieve you of any concerns you might have about the tests.

CHAPTER CHECKLIST

1. On October 1, 1994 the Mammography Quality and Safety Act (MQSA) implemented by the Food and Drug Administration went into effect. The American College of Radiology has been approved as the accrediting body to insure specific standards of compliance for mammography facilities. You still may want to call your mammogram site to confirm that they have met the standards issued under the MQSA. They will be able to answer other questions that you may have such as: How many mammograms do they perform in a week? month? What is their policy regarding results? Are they immediate or must you wait days for results?

2. What other tests, such as ultrasound, are performed at that site? If a board-certified site is at a hospital, ask what they have for diagnostic equipment for other tests and scans. If it is a first-rate facility you will be returning for future tests.

3. Inquire if there are any specific instructions that you must follow prior to your test, such as limiting medications or food intake.

4. Mentally prepare yourself for the tests or scans. Don't be frightened or anticipate the worst. Tests and scans are important tools necessary to an accurate diagnosis. Take a

friend if that will provide diversion or keep you relaxed. Personally, I was more comfortable alone, but most women are pleased to have the comfort of a friend or relative.

5. Dress simply and appropriately; wear comfortable, easy-to-remove clothing. Unless you have appointments prior to or after tests, sweat suits are perfect for comfort and warmth. Keep a jacket or wrap handy in the waiting room and in the diagnostic rooms. The machines must be maintained in a climate-controlled environment.

6. At each step in the procedures you are likely to find delays. Bring reading, paperwork, needlepoint, or something that you can do while you wait for the technician to prepare the film or equipment. You will also wait after the test while the technician examines the exposed film or monitor for clarity.

7. Organize yourself. Bring checks, credit cards, insurance-reimbursement forms completed with your basic personal information, and insurance card. You will be able to bring your purse or briefcase with you into the room where you will be having your test.

8. When you are in the facility, look for the certificate of accreditation and also look for a dated sticker on the equipment. This is added insurance that they are in compliance with certification regulations.

9. Ask for the results of the scans to be sent to your doctor. Also, ask for a written copy of the evaluation of the scans for your files and a duplicate copy of any photographs pertinent to your diagnosis.

CHAPTER 5

....

Medical Procedures

Rebecca: The medical examination by your doctor has confirmed your suspicions, and the lump now needs further investigation. You have had the supporting diagnostic procedures; a mammogram and possibly an ultrasound or another test that has also proven that this lump might be more than a fluid-filled cyst. The reality that this might be breast cancer begins to sink in. I remember a feeling of being swept along, almost powerlessly, with the process of getting this lump diagnosed. First the doctor, next the mammogram, then the ultrasound. What next?

Dr. Petrek: Only a biopsy can give you reliable results about whether this lump is a breast cancer or not. There are several types of biopsies, but the definitive biopsy procedure is the excisional or surgical biopsy. Since this is a surgical procedure I would recommend that you seek a general surgeon who has had significant breast experience or, better yet, a breast surgeon specialist. Your doctor may be willing to recommend one or two breast surgeons in your area to perform this procedure.

Rebecca: Even though a large percent of lumps that are biopsied prove to be benign, you want the best surgeon you can find that practices at the best hospital available. Many women that I have spoken with fail to have a breast surgeon perform their biopsy. Rather, they have a general surgeon remove what is a routine lump that probably is not malignant. The problem is that if the lump proves to be malignant, enough surrounding breast tissue may not be taken the first time and the surgeon may have to recut the original site to take additional breast tissue for more complete pathological examination. It is better to be sure that the surgeon performing the biopsy, and the hospital, are experienced in dealing with cancer. Chapter 9, Second Opinion Consultations, will give you guidelines on researching specialists and hospitals. In other words, in choosing your surgeon and the hospital facilities, assume your lump is malignant until it is proven otherwise.

The surgeon will perform the same type of physical examination of your breasts as your family doctor or your gynecologist did. He may then want to first perform a needle biopsy or needle aspiration to eliminate the possibility that your lump may be a fluid-filled cyst and not breast cancer at all. If the fluid does not drain and the lump does not disappear, then a surgical biopsy will probably be recommended.

Needle Biopsy

Dr. Petrek: A needle biopsy can be the first procedure done by the breast surgeon specialist when confronted with a lump. The surgeon will not know whether the lump is a cancer or not, and the needle biopsy is a good procedure for learning about the nature of the lump. The needle biopsy is quick, simple, and not painful; there is no cut into the breast with this procedure and it is performed in the doctor's office. The area is cleaned, and a thin, hollow needle is inserted through the skin and into the breast lump. The fluid and tissue from the lump are drawn into the hollow needle and then prepared on a slide for laboratory analysis. Pathological evaluation of the tissue and fluid can determine normal cells or can reveal abnormal or "atypical" cells.

Rebecca: Waiting for the biopsy results can be frustrating and frightening; be certain to ask the surgeon how long it will take to receive the results. Some laboratories are overloaded, and it is not unusual to wait an agonizing week or ten days. Meanwhile, what happens to the lump?

Dr. Petrek: While the presence of lumps can cause a great deal of anxiety, remember that a large percentage, 85 percent, of all biopsied breast lumps are benign. The needle biopsy procedure itself can be reassuring because often the lump is a fluid-filled cyst that drains when it is punctured and completely disappears. If no fluid is drawn from the lump or it does not completely disappear, then there must be a definitive biopsy.

Rebecca: The needle biopsy sounds gruesome but it really isn't, and it is a useful tool to the surgeon in determining who may need a more extensive biopsy. However, two factors are extremely important to consider when having a needle biopsy. The first is the skill of the doctor performing the needle biopsy. Ideally, it should be a breast surgeon specialist. Under no circumstances do you want the doctor guiding the needle to miss the cancer and produce a negative laboratory analysis when in fact cancer cells are present.

Second, the quality of the laboratory that handles your breast tissue is critical. So much of cancer diagnosis and treatment decisions are based on the pathology of your tumor. Question your doctor about the labs he uses and make certain that it is a laboratory experienced in providing the appropriate tests associated with cancer. The procedure takes only minutes and the cost of the needle biopsy should be in the range of $150 to $400, including the fee of the breast surgeon specialist. The laboratory fees may run from $75 to $120.

The Stereotactic Core Biopsy

Dr. Petrek: The stereotactic core biopsy is a procedure used almost exclusively on abnormalities that are seen on a mammogram but are not felt upon manual examination. After a mammogram discovers a small lump or calcifications that might mean cancer is present, a computerized three-dimensional X ray finds the exact location of the questionable tissue. The doctor then uses a needle guided by the computer and takes a sample of the lump or suspicious breast tissue for pathological analysis. The large-core biopsy produces a cylinder 2 mm in diameter by 20 mm in length.

There are advantages to using the stereotactic biopsy. First, there is no residual scar from a surgical incision; second, it is not painful and only local anesthesia is needed; and third, the procedure is done on an outpatient basis and therefore less expensive. The stereotactic biopsy equipment can also be used with a fine needle instead of a core needle although that procedure is not as common.

Rebecca: The core-biopsy procedure was not available when I had my breast cancer but today most cancer centers and large university hospitals are using the core biopsy for certain women with suspicious mammograms. The procedure takes about one half an hour and can cost from $1,500 to $2,000. This may seem expensive, but the cost of the equipment, the training and skill of the doctor using the sophisticated equipment make the core biopsy a costly procedure.

The Surgical Biopsy

Dr. Petrek: The surgical or excisional biopsy is the most commonly used procedure in a definitive breast cancer diagnosis. If there is a lump of a suspicious nature or if the results of a needle biopsy prove "atypical" or not normal, then a surgical biopsy is usually recommended. The excisional biopsy is a surgical procedure performed under local anesthesia or monitored sedation. Only rarely is general anesthesia ever required.

The surgeon will make a small incision on the breast near the site, with the length dependent upon the lump size. The lump is removed with some surrounding breast tissue, sometimes referred to as margins. The lump and the tissue can be subjected to a frozen-section analysis, or rapid section, although it is becoming common to not request a frozen section and to wait for the definitive results of the permanent section. For lumps that are small there may not be enough tissue to perform a frozen section analysis. The tissue is frozen so that a slice of the lump can be immediately examined under a microscope. This analysis can determine whether your lump is cancerous or not.

The frozen section diagnosis is not usually different from the permanent section analysis that will be performed on the lump in the laboratory. (A detailed explanation on pathology follows in chapter 6.) When you are alert, your surgeon can give you the results on whether the lump is malignant or not based on the frozen section if performed.

In some instances the lump is large but the surgeon may not think it is a tumor. In that case an incisional biopsy may be performed. This involves the taking of a portion of the lump for pathological analysis. In the case of an incisional biopsy or excisional biopsy, both surgeries are performed in the same medical setting with the same presurgical requirements.

Rebecca: This excisional or incisional biopsy procedure can be performed in the outpatient or ambulatory surgery floor of a hospital, in a medical clinic, or in a doctor's office if it is surgically equipped. If you intend to have this procedure performed in a hospital on an outpatient basis, you will be required to take some routine tests such as a chest X ray, blood workup, and electrocardiogram depending on your age, just as you would for any other type of surgery. If you live relatively near the hospital, you can schedule these tests a few days in advance of your biopsy.

The surgical biopsy procedure will be done by a breast surgeon specialist or a general surgeon experienced in breast treatment. It would rarely be done by your gynecologist or your family doctor although both of them should be consulted when you are looking for a doctor to perform the surgical breast biopsy. Obviously you will want a surgeon who is experienced in doing breast biopsies and ideally one whose specialty is breast surgery.

Your surgeon should explain to you what the procedure involves, how much breast tissue he will remove in addition to the lump, and when you can expect the results of the pathological analysis of the lump.

You will also want him or her to be practicing at a quality medical facility. While statistics indicate that a large percentage, 85 percent, of all biopsied breast lumps prove to be benign, you want to place yourself in the most competent hands you can find. The surgical biopsy, even on an outpatient basis, requires the use of surgical facilities and is therefore expensive. Including the presurgical tests, the surgeon's fee, the anesthesiologist, the hospital, and the lab fees, the cost of the surgical biopsy can be $4,000 to $5,000.

Incidentally, today, a woman rarely signs a surgical consent form that allows her doctor to perform additional breast surgery based on the results of a biopsy procedure. We are fortunate that we will no longer have a simple biopsy procedure done and then wake up from the anesthesia having lost a breast. Thanks to pioneering breast cancer advocates, the lumpectomy procedure is almost always separate from any additional breast surgery.

I still discover, however, women who have wanted to have a mastectomy while still under the effects of anesthesia if their lump proved to be cancerous. Many of those women have regretted their premature decision. A friend of my mother's, Jeanice, a stunning woman in her late sixties, felt that if her lump was cancerous she wanted the breast removed. After the mastectomy her doctor told her that the lump was small and that she would be fine. Even now, several years later, she feels that she acted hastily. If she had taken more time for another consultation and some investigation, she might have chosen breast conservation instead.

Fortunately, most surgeons recommend the two-step approach to diagnosing breast lumps and will refuse to perform additional surgery until the woman has had an opportunity to think through her diagnosis.

CHAPTER CHECKLIST

1. The mammogram or another test may not conclusively indicate cancer, but the evidence suggests that the lump must be pathologically examined. Have your doctor recommend one or two breast surgeon specialists for you to call. Ask him how often he refers patients to them; where they practice; and at what hospitals they have privileges. Be alert to the network of doctors practicing at the same hospital.
2. Follow the instructions in chapters 8 and 9 for investigating the surgeon and hospital. If you are at high risk for breast cancer, you will want to be at a hospital experienced at dealing with malignant biopsies.
3. The percentages indicate that most breast lumps are be-

nign. Take comfort in this knowledge, but do your investigative research in the event that you are in the minority.

4. Select the surgeon and make the call. Briefly explain your situation to schedule the appointment as quickly as possible.

5. Prepare a list of questions for the surgeon. Will he do a needle biopsy? How long will the results take? Will the results determine whether a surgical biopsy is needed? Will a surgical biopsy be done regardless of the results of the needle biopsy?

6. Have him explain in detail how he proceeds with biopsies. What type of anesthesia does he use? Local, monitored sedation, general or other? Where will the incision be? How large will it be? Will he remove additional breast tissue or margins for evaluation? Will an immediate frozen section analysis be done? Can the laboratory do the up-to-date tumor tests in the event of malignancy? What are they? Will you have the results at the hospital that day? When?

7. Does he have a nurse or someone in his office with whom you can speak when scheduling the hospital, the presurgery prep tests, additional tests and scans, or answer other questions that might come up? How available will he or she be for additional consultations?

CHAPTER 6

....

Pathological Diagnosis

Rebecca: We know that 85 percent of breast lumps that are biopsied are benign. But, that also means that there are still 15 percent of breast lumps that are malignant. I was shocked when the surgeon told me that I was among the minority and that my lump was a breast cancer. What does this mean?

Dr. Petrek: During the surgical biopsy your lump was removed, a small piece was frozen and then sliced for immediate microscopic analysis. It was the result of this frozen-section pathological analysis that determined whether the lump was cancer or not. For small lumps, especially those found mammographically, a frozen section is not taken and the tissue is evaluated in a permanent section pathological analysis.

Rebecca: In the years prior to the separation of the diagnostic surgery and the treatment surgery, the surgeon decided then whether or not to remove the breast and the underarm lymph nodes. The woman was still under the effects of general anesthesia and the additional surgery was performed on the basis of one brief examination of the tissue.

Dr. Petrek: Yes. Now we feel that a diagnosis determined by the frozen section analysis method, while almost always accurate, is not as definitive as an examination by permanent section pathology. In some cases, a frozen section analysis on a small lump could be counterproductive due to the size of the lump and may not produce the best results. The type of surgery you will have and the treatment of your cancer will depend on the composition of your tumor.

The more reliable preparation of a tumor specimen is to have it enclosed in wax and then thinly sliced onto prepared slides for further microscopic examination. This is known as a permanent section analysis or permanent paraffin technique. This is the preferred method because the staining properties are better and the tumor tissue is more precisely defined. The permanent section slides take from three to seven days to prepare. Incidentally, the laboratory is required to keep your tumor in a paraffin block for several years.

When the pathologist looks at a slice of your tumor under a microscope, he is searching for malignant breast cells, which are quite different from normal breast cells. As cancerous cells multiply they develop different characteristics that the pathologist can see, which are unlike normal breast tissue cells. This is known as differentiation.

He also looks for invasion or infiltration, or the presence of cancer cells invading into healthy tissue. Healthy cells multiply where they began and do not spread. Benign tumor cells push against healthy tissue and do not invade it. Even a tumor that contains cells that look benign can be diagnosed as malignant if cells can be seen invading surrounding breast tissue.

The pathologist will want to determine if the tumor has the ability to metastasize or move from the breast through the lymph vessels or blood vessels to another location or organ in the body. The pathologist can tell from the microscopic picture of a cancer cell that it may be capable of moving to another part of the body. Remember, breast cancer in the breast does not kill women, it is when breast cancer spreads to vital organs such as the lungs, liver, or bone that the disease can ultimately prove fatal.

Rebecca: The pathologist can perform several other tests on the biopsied breast lump that can provide important information. The most common laboratory test that should be performed on a biopsied breast lump is called an estrogen receptor assay (ERA) and progesterone receptor assay (PRA). Can you explain what this is?

Dr. Petrek: We know that our bodies produce the hormones estrogen and progesterone. These are substances produced internally that regulate many of our bodily functions such as our sexual organs, menstrual cycles, and menopause. The breasts are very sensitive to these hormones. An estrogen receptor test (ERA) and the progesterone receptor test (PRA) will determine to what extent your breast cancer is influenced by hormones. These tests measure the receptor proteins that bind to the estrogen and progesterone and can be present in the cells of a breast cancer tumor. Approximately 50 percent of breast cancers contain estrogen and progesterone receptors which can promote tumor growth in the presence of hormones. Those tumors that are graded as having estrogen-progesterone receptors are labelled ER–PR positive and the other 50 percent of breast tumors that do not have significant estrogen-progesterone receptors are called ER–PR negative. The results of this test can help determine whether you might be a good candidate for antihormone treatment or possibly chemotherapy following your breast cancer surgery.

Rebecca: Are there other tests which the more sophisticated hospitals and laboratories may use to complete the pathology picture of breast tumors?

Dr. Petrek: Yes. A DNA flow cytometry test may be performed on her tumor. This is a laboratory test that measures the quantity and quality of DNA in breast cancer cells and then compares them with healthy breast cells. This test is sometimes helpful in determining the rate of growth of a tumor and its ability to spread to other parts of the body. The results give your doctor necessary information to evaluate your risks of recurrence and can help in determining whether to treat you with chemotherapy, especially in women with negative lymph nodes. Many laboratories are not equipped to perform this test and it is expensive, $250 to $400, so you will want to ask your doctor if this is appropriate for you.

Rebecca: In May of 1988 the National Cancer Institute issued an advisory to 13,000 doctors and the media regarding treatment recommendations for women who have had breast cancer and whose lymph nodes were analyzed and found to be clear of cancer. This is considered node-negative breast cancer. This "clinical alert" suggested that all node-negative women, with the exception of those women whose cancers were confined to a milk duct or those women with invasive tumors less than one centimeter in size, should consider adjuvant therapy. Adjuvant or additional therapy could be either chemotherapy, in the form of a combination of anticancer drugs for a limited period of time, or hormone therapy, in which a woman receives in pill form a medication to prevent estrogen from promoting possible cancer cells. My surgery was in June of 1988 and the "clinical alert" without doubt was instrumental to my receiving chemotherapy and hormone therapy.

Dr. Petrek: This advisory has changed the way doctors treat node-negative women, and treatment decisions are based largely on the pathology of the breast tumor and pathological diagnosis of the lymph nodes. The importance of the role of the pathologist and the quality of the laboratory that actually performs these tests has great bearing on your subsequent treatment. Decisions regarding the extent of your cancer, the type of surgery you will need, and the follow-up treatment recommended to you are largely determined by the size and composition of your tumor. Complete and thorough analysis of your tumor is critical to a successful cure of breast cancer. A good breast surgeon recognizes the importance of the pathology performed on his patients and places great faith in the laboratory analysis.

Rebecca: Some hospitals have in-house laboratory facilities, but in some rural hospitals the tissue is sent out of state to a distant lab and it can take weeks to obtain the results. Sarah, a young woman that I met in Vermont, had a breast biopsy and the hospital laboratory had sent it out for analysis. She waited nearly three weeks for the results.

Breast biopsies are inconvenient at best and when you have a job and family that depend on you this delay can create tremendous anxiety. I have heard many complaints from women who have asked to have their tumor sent to another laboratory for analysis and their surgeons never followed through on their request. As a result, they were left with incomplete tissue specimens and a worthless piece of paper that describes very little about the pathology of her tumor. A woman needs to be assertive in demanding that her tumor be appropriately analyzed. Acceptable is not good enough when determining the quality of the pathology.

CHAPTER CHECKLIST

1. Question the surgeon performing your biopsy on the quality of the laboratory that will be analyzing your lump. Is it a commercial lab or a large hospital pathology department? Who is the chief pathologist? Are the results timely? When can they be expected? Will they prepare the tissue slides? Will they write a detailed report on your tumor?

2. If the tumor is malignant, can the lab perform the latest tests? The estrogen receptor assay (ERA) and the progesterone receptor assay (PRA)? The DNA flow cytometry?

3. Will the doctor send your tumor specimen to another hospital or pathology lab of your choosing? How should you arrange this?

CHAPTER 7

....

The Cancer Worksheet

Rebecca: Cancer. The word alone can produce a variety of reactions in different people. For some people it means death, for other people it can mean pain and suffering, but in everyone the word generates fear. Cancer can strike any person. You can be young or old, rich or poor, of any race, creed, or color.

Dr. Petrek: Since the turn of the century the medical profession and most of the supporting medical organizations and associations have been engaged in research and study to control and cure cancer. The National Cancer Institute, the National Institutes of Health, the American Cancer Society, and many independent educational and medical institutions have spent billions of dollars in an effort to discover a cure. The goal of these institutions is to make cancer a disease of the past in the same way that diseases such as polio and smallpox have been eradicated. Indeed, great strides have been made in understanding the biology and growth of cancer both in the laboratory and through the use of patient clinical trials. Improvements in surgery, radiation, and chemotherapy provide the patient with greater quality of treatment with fewer adverse side effects.

Rebecca: As significant as these medical advances are, there is no substitute for the intimate knowledge a woman has of her own body to detect an early breast cancer. In short, we can do more for our own breast health by having regularly scheduled screening mammography, performing breast self-examination monthly, and by having regular breast examinations by a doctor.

Dr. Petrek: That is right. Most women have secondhand knowledge of breast cancer, and many confusing factors support public misconception about the disease. This could be the reason that keeps women from being diligent about examining their own bodies.

People in general tend to think of cancer as just one disease, but, in fact, it is more than a hundred different diseases with just as many different characteristics. Breast cancer is just one of many types of cancers, but it is one of the most unpredictable. We have suspicions about what can cause breast cancer, but we really don't know why certain cells change from healthy and normal to become a cancer.

To increase our understanding of breast cancer, it is important to study the risk factors associated with disease development: who might possibly get breast cancer and why. No one specific cause determines who will get breast cancer. There are, however, documented risk patterns that could increase a woman's chances of developing breast cancer. Lifestyle profiles, such as your diet, your personality type, and certain environmental exposures may increase the possibility of a breast cancer diagnosis.

Rebecca: I observed that in the course of my own diagnosis of breast cancer most doctors, and even some technicians, ask for a personal medical history. Some doctors ask for information in great detail, while others are concerned with specific aspects of your lifestyle or medical history. In this chapter we are going to build what we call a Cancer Worksheet. If we discuss briefly the risk patterns of those women who do get cancer, examine the few specific lifestyle profiles that we can control, and relate them to your own life, we can create a format for charting your own medical history.

There are many reasons why it is important to review the risks associated with breast cancer. On a personal level, it is difficult for many women to deal with a breast cancer diagnosis. When they stop to reflect on what this diagnosis means, many women blame themselves or their lifestyle for the fact that they have cancer. They feel they must have done something wrong to have brought on this disease. I admit that I felt that way, and I also knew that some of my lifestyle habits were less than healthy.

In reviewing the list of risk factors we will see that they are as varied as our own lives. Some risks may possibly apply to you, while others may be irrelevant for you. It is important to keep in mind when you read the risk patterns that some risks are well-documented and known to promote breast cancer and other risks have not had enough careful study to firmly convince the medical experts that they may in fact contribute to a breast cancer diagnosis.

However, you should be aware of all potential risks. Clearly there are factors that are beyond your control, while there are some lifestyle changes that you can adopt immediately to improve your health and reduce your risk for breast cancer.

Dr. Petrek: From a professional perspective, doctors recognize that all women are unique individuals who come to them with lifelong medical histories and habits, both good and bad. They are looking for any and all information that will help them to make an appropriate diagnosis of the patient's breast cancer and suggest treatment that can cure her of breast cancer.

Rebecca: With the completion of the Cancer Worksheet you will have at hand the information that might be requested from the medical professionals as you seek a breast cancer diagnosis. During this stressful period you will be organized, you will be able to communicate fully and cooperate with the doctor, and you will spare yourself the additional anxiety of having to repeatedly re-create your medical history for each of the professionals you see.

Risk Patterns

Dr. Petrek: In the following pages I want you to review the risks and honestly consider whether you might fit into the profile. All women are at significant risk for getting breast cancer. Some women, however, are considered to be at higher risk than others and should have more frequent examinations and take whatever preventive procedures possible to protect themselves. You should be aware of risk patterns that may apply to you, but keep in mind that the statistics stated are subjective with variables that affect outcomes. Statistics should be viewed as rough estimates that may or may not be applicable to you.

The risk factors are listed in order of importance. Age and family history are by far the most predictive, while the remaining risk factors are documented to increase the incidence of breast cancer, they are much less important.

1. *Age:* The incidence of breast cancer increases with age and women are living longer. According to the American Cancer Society 75 percent of all breast cancers occur in women over the age of 50. And National Cancer Institute studies indicate that 75 percent of women who do develop breast cancer have no serious risk factors other than age.

The number of cases of young women developing breast cancer increases almost yearly, it seems. Just a few years ago most breast cancers occurred in women over 50 years old and half of those occurred in women over the age of 65. Now there are increasing numbers of women in their forties diagnosed with breast cancer. One theory is that more breast cancers are detected earlier because mammography screening is more prevalent today. Premenopausal breast cancer patients, however, tend to have faster growing, more aggressive tumors than older women.

2. *Family History:* A woman whose mother or sister had breast cancer has a greater risk than that of other women. The closer the relative, the younger the age of diagnosis, and if the cancer occurred in both breasts can mean even more increased risk. However, 75 to 85 percent of women diagnosed with breast cancer have no family history of the disease. Researchers are currently working to characterize the gene on a particular chromosome that is known to cause 5 to 7 percent of all breast cancer cases. With a genetic predisposition you may also have a breast cancer at the age of the relative or possibly earlier.

3. *Menstrual History:* Because estrogen production increases at the start of menstruation, women with long menstrual histories—early menstruation through a late menopause—are at increased risk. The age at which menstruation begins has dropped steadily over the years, from age 17 to age 12 in the last two centuries. A woman who began her first menstrual period at age 12 has a greater risk of developing breast cancer than a woman whose first period started at age 15. Share your female, breast, and reproductive history with your daughters so that they can chart their own medical histories. At the other end of the age range, a woman has a greater risk of developing breast cancer the older she is when she enters menopause. Conversely, early menopause can reduce the risk because our breasts are exposed to less estrogen over time.

4. *Childbearing History:* Women who have no children or women who have delayed having their first child until after the age of 30 seem to be at greater risk, 17 to 20 percent, for developing breast cancer. For instance, a woman who had her first child when she was thirty is at greater risk of developing breast cancer than a woman who had her first child in her early twenties. In other words, this is a minor increase, not even double the risk.

Those who took the drug diethylstilbestrol (DES) to prevent miscarriage when they were pregnant are at increased risk. The millions of women who took the high-dose older birth control pills for any duration may also be at risk. The millions of women who have taken the middle-dose birth control pill and in particular the low-dose birth control pill for a long duration may be at lower risk, probably because ovarian function is suppressed and there is a lower hormone environment.

5. *Breast Feeding:* Women who have babies at an early age, prior to age 30, and breast-feed their babies for six months or longer tend to reduce their risk of getting premenopausal breast cancer. Breast-feeding seems to offer some protection against getting breast cancer, at least before menopause.

6. *Previous Breast or Other Type of Cancer:* A woman who has developed cancer in one breast has a 25 percent probability of developing a second cancer in the same breast or in the other breast. This could also be true of women with previous uterine cancer. This seems to be true, although it is difficult to assign any meaningful statistics, because each case of breast cancer is unique to the individual woman.

7. *Benign or Fibrocystic Breast Disease:* Fibrocystic or breast cyst changes do not predict a higher risk of breast cancer, whether the diagnosis was made by physical examination or biopsy. However, about 5 percent of benign (usually so-called fibrocystic) biopsies will also show "atypical" cells, and these 5 percent of women are at higher risk for breast cancer.

8. *Body Estrogen Production and/or Synthetic Estrogen Intake:* The hormone estrogen is known to stimulate the growth of breast tissue and therefore could promote the growth of any breast cancer cells that are present within breast tissue. Our bodies produce the hormone estrogen during our child-bearing years. The ovaries are the greatest source of estrogen production in premenopausal women, but the adrenal glands and to a lesser degree our own body fat also produce estrogen. In fact, at the turn of the twentieth century the ovaries were removed in women who had breast cancer, and this surgery was one of the earliest treatments for breast cancer.

There is increasing evidence, although not formally conclusive according to a recent article in the *New England Journal of Medicine,* that taking synthetic estrogens can add to the risk of breast cancer in some women. Women who take estrogen or estrogen and progestin combination therapy for many years for relief of menopausal symptoms should be aware that they may be at increased risk, possibly from 10 to 30 percent, for developing breast cancer. Because estrogen therapy can produce excellent benefits, such as reducing the risk of heart disease and keeping osteoporosis in check, each woman should discuss these risks with her doctor.

9. *Exposure to Radiation:* There is increased risk to women who have had breast, neck, or chest radiation at a young age, such as in their teenage years. The younger the age, the greater the risk, no matter what the exposure. Some women will and do use radiation risk as an excuse to avoid the mammogram and other necessary X rays. In the normal course of our lives it is highly unlikely that we will develop cancer as a result of routine diagnostic X rays. And, in the case of the mammogram, the benefits of early breast cancer detection by mammography far outweigh the insignificant risk of radiation.

10. *Geography:* According to reports from the Centers for

Disease Control, the rate of death from breast cancer is highest in the Northern half of the U.S. The lowest rates tended to be in the South or Southwest. We don't really know why, but this could be due to the greater degree of industrialization, pollution, and environmental toxins. There are great variations in the breast cancer rates of other countries.

11. *Ethnic Origin:* Cancer in the breast is the most common malignant tumor in women. According to the American Cancer Society, 182,000 women will be diagnosed in 1994 with breast cancer. Of those new cases, approximately 10 percent will be among black Americans and 3 percent among minority Americans. There have been slightly higher incidences of breast cancer across the board in white American women and African-American women in recent years.

12. *Lifestyle—Environment:* Lengthy exposure to toxic chemical and environmental substances have been known to increase the risk of certain cancers and possibly breast cancer as well. These may be in the form of pesticides, toxic substances, asbestos, electromagnetic fields from power lines, contaminated water, and certain industrial carcinogens in the workplace. However, early references of breast cancer were hieroglyphic translations attributed to the Egyptian physician Imhotep around 3000 B.C. and recorded in the Edwin Smith Papyrus. Throughout history, long before industrialization, references were made to breast cancer.

13. *Lifestyle—Personality:* There has been increasing speculation about the link between personality type and women who get breast cancer. Certain traits—such as trying to be a perfectionist, suppressing anger, chronic hostility, aggressiveness, inability to cope with stress, low self-esteem, feeling overwhelmed by responsibilities—can contribute to increased risk of various diseases and possibly breast cancer. Studies are inconclusive, but some doctors believe that breast cancer might be influenced by personality type or stress.

14. *Lifestyle—Diet and Nutrition:* Considerable research has been carried out on the correlation between diet and breast cancer, with a wide range of results. If you are careless about your diet and consume large portions of animal and vegetable fats and sugars and fail to regulate the quantity and quality of your food choices, your body could be nutritionally deficient and you could be at higher risk for developing breast cancer. About 20–30 percent of breast cancers may have a possible connection with a diet high in fat. Although no diet can cure breast cancer, there are definite health benefits to maintaining a balanced, sensible diet that is high in fruits, vegetables, and whole grains. You must also eat a minimum of fat, animal proteins, and calories. A preventive diet could possibly offer us some protection against breast cancer.

15. *Lifestyle—Alcohol and Tobacco:* These are two unhealthy habits not always associated with breast cancer risk. There have been increased discussions, however, on the link between alcohol and breast cancer. Most doctors recommend that you limit your alcohol consumption to less than one or two drinks a day. No link is known between tobacco and breast cancer, but there is no reason to smoke.

16. *Lifestyle—Exercise:* We know that daily exercise is the single most important thing we can do to maintain our bodies, but a possible relationship may exist between exercise and reduced cancer risk. Being active helps to reduce body fat. And lower fat means a reduction of estrogen hormones that may contribute to breast cancer. Moderate, daily exercise will help you to maintain your normal body weight.

17. *Lifestyle—Regular Medical Maintenance:* If you do not engage in regular preventive medical maintenance, you could increase your risk of not finding an early, potentially curable breast cancer. You should have regular physical checkups and yearly pelvic and breast examinations, including a Pap smear, by a gynecologist. You should be on an age-appropriate schedule of mammograms; the American Cancer Society recommends a first screening by age 40, a mammogram every 1 to 2 years between age 40 and 49, and an annual mammogram over age 50. And you should be performing regular monthly breast self-examinations. There is no substitute for seeing experienced doctors who objectively watch over your health.

Rebecca: Dr. Petrek, after reading the list of risk patterns it becomes clear why more women are being diagnosed with breast cancer. Based on the breadth of risks it is no wonder that we feel threatened by it.

About the Cancer Worksheet

On the next few pages you will find a sample format for the types of questions you may be asked to answer in each of your medical consultations. It is more than any one doctor requires. It is invaluable, however, to have the information in one central place so that any doctor can select the information appropriate to his specialty. The information is arranged in five categories. The first section is Technical Information about you, your spouse, your primary care doctors, and your insurers.

The second section requests your Personal Medical History. This will take some time and thought, especially if you have had any serious illnesses.

The third section asks for the Family Medical History. You may want to contact a parent or relative to help you complete this section.

The fourth section concerns your Feminine History. This is divided into four sections: reproductive, gynecologic, preventive, and breast histories. This section may also take time to complete and you can have your primary-care doctor's nurse or secretary help you.

The fifth and last section deals with your Lifestyle History.

Based on the review of the risk and lifestyle patterns you should be able to honestly respond to any questions that may be asked of you. Different doctors practicing in different specialties will be interested in different parts of this worksheet. To save time and get the most out of your office visit or consultation, complete the worksheet to the best of your ability and devote the maximum amount of time with the doctor for discussions about your breast cancer.

CHAPTER CHECKLIST

1. Do not be needlessly frightened by the risk patterns that may contribute to breast cancer. Use them as a basis for analyzing your medical history and for reducing your current risks and improving your personal lifestyle habits.

2. Accept this diagnosis as a learning experience, a crash course in cancer, a challenging opportunity to take positive action for your life.

3. You may at first question why you are bothering to complete this form but it will be apparent to you immediately at your first meeting with a doctor. This is important information for the doctor but can be a nuisance for you to have to repeat to each professional you come in contact with.

4. Keep several copies of this form with you for all tests and appointments. You won't be sorry.

CANCER WORKSHEET

1. Technical Information

Name: Employer:
Address: Address:

Telephone (home):
Telephone (office):   Telephone:

Social Security #

Marital Status: Single: Married: Divorced: Widowed: Separated:

Insurance Company:
  Address:
  Policy or Group Number:
  Policy Holder Name:
  Address:
  Relationship to Policy Holder:

Family physician: Gynecologist:
  Address: Address:
  Telephone: Telephone:

Other Referring Doctor:
  Address:
  Telephone:

2. Personal Medical History

Date of Birth: Age: Where?
How would you describe your general health?
Do you have an annual physical with a primary care physician?
When was your last physical exam?
What are your vitals signs:
Weight: Blood pressure:
Height: Cholesterol:
How many times did you see a doctor this year?   For what?
Have you had or do you currently have any serious illnesses?
What?   When?
Have you had major surgery?
For what?   When?
Have you had any other hospitalizations?
For what?   When?
Have you ever had radiation treatment?   For what?

Are you currently taking any medications?
What?   Dosage?   How long?
Do you take vitamins?   What type?   Dosage?
Did you have any serious childhood illnesses?
What?   When?

3. Family Medical History

What is your racial background (optional)?
Are your immediate ancestors living in the U.S.?
What diseases or medical conditions affected your immediate family?
Heart disease   High blood pressure   Other
Heart attack   Diabetes
Has anyone in your immediate family had cancer?   Age?
Ovarian   Lung   Other
Uterine   Prostate
Did your mother or sister have breast cancer?   Age?
One or both breasts?   How was it treated?

4. Feminine History

Reproductive:
Do you have children?   What are their ages?
How old were you when you had your first child?
Was it a normal delivery?   Were other deliveries normal?
Did you breast feed?   How long?
Did you have any abortions or miscarriages?

Gynecologic:
At what age did you begin menstruation?
Have you ever taken birth control pills?   When?
Have you used any other form of birth control?   What?
Do you have a history of infertility?
Have you taken drugs for infertility?
Are you menopausal?   At what age did menstruation cease?
Do you have any menopausal symptoms?
   Hot flashes?   Night sweats?   Weight gain?
   Mood swings?   Depression?   Vaginal dryness?
Have you had any menstrual bleeding in the last year?
Have you ever or do you currently take estrogen?
In what form?   What dosage?
Have you ever had a hysterectomy?   When?
Did you have removal of the uterus?   Ovaries?
Have you ever had: Pelvic Ultrasound?   Endometrial Biopsy?

Preventive:
Do you see a gynecologist?   How often?
Does he/she examine your breasts at each visit?
Does he/she give you a pelvic examination?
Does he/she do a Pap smear?   How often?
When was your last mammogram?
Prior mammograms?

Breast:
Do you have benign or fibrocystic breast disease?
Have you had a previous breast biopsy?   When?
  What were the results?
Have you had a previous breast cancer?   When?
  What form of treatment did you have?
    Surgery?   Chemotherapy?
    Radiation?   Hormone Therapy?
Have you ever had: Bone scan?   Breast ultrasound?

5. Lifestyle History

Is your typical diet considered adequate? Is is low in fat?
Do you eat sweets?   Drink caffeine?   Snack?   Binge/purge?
Do you consume alcohol?
How much?   How often?
Do you smoke?   How much?   For how long?
Do you exercise regularly?   What type?   How often?
Do you have great weight fluctuations?
Do you consider yourself overweight?
What type of personality do you have?   Passive/Aggressive?
Are you under constant stress, either at home or on the job?
Are there any environmental factors that might contribute to
cancer?
Have you ever been exposed to certain chemicals or excessive
radiation?

PART THREE

Investigation

CHAPTER 8

....

Second Opinion Consultations

Rebecca: To summarize where you are in the process of a breast cancer diagnosis, let us review what has happened up to this point. The lump that you discovered or that was found as a result of mammography has confirmed your suspicions that breast cancer might be a possibility. You should have had the appropriate diagnostic procedures, followed by the medical and surgical procedures necessary in confirming a potential breast cancer. The pathological diagnosis is complete, and the definitive results confirm that you do have breast cancer. What now? You have many questions, but who do you ask? What can you do? How can you find the information that you will need to make a decision about how to proceed next?

A great deal of information and many resources are available to the woman confronted with a breast cancer diagnosis. The subject has been written about from a variety of perspectives ranging from the very personal to the highly technical. Unfortunately, such information is not always readily available when we need it.

There are two good methods for accumulating the specific information that you will need to make a confident decision about adequate and appropriate treatment for your breast cancer. First, effective communication and interaction with the medical professionals whom you see should give you access to the latest information and treatment options available. Second, you can support that information with discussions and written materials from the many health care resource centers, agencies, and organizations dedicated to breast cancer research and treatment.

In Part Five we have compiled a Database list of sources and resources to assist a woman in her search for as much information as she is willing to digest. It will be useful in providing supplemental material on breast cancer as well as names and locations of specialists and hospitals.

Preparing a List of Specialists

Dr. Petrek: As a woman takes positive action in getting her breast lump diagnosed either as benign or, unfortunately, as a malignant breast tumor, she begins to realize that she has accumulated a great deal of knowledge about breast cancer. Each doctor, nurse, social worker, or technician has provided specific details about procedures needed to evaluate her breast lump. These people are all professionals and want you to understand what is happening to you at each step in determining an accurate diagnosis. They are your best source for up-to-date information on breast cancer. Communicate and confide in them. The information that you gather during the confirmation process is just the beginning of a storehouse of knowledge that you will need to make an informed decision about how to treat your breast cancer.

Rebecca: It becomes evident that you will have to make a great many choices regarding your breast cancer. The treatment is more complicated than you imagined. There is no one standard treatment for breast cancer and you may get contradictory recommendations about what surgeries and treatments may be best for you. It becomes clear that you must pull together a list of specialists to consider for second and third opinion consultations. The examination results from the second and third opinion physicians you meet should add to and clarify the information you have already received.

Your doctor is probably not going to volunteer to consult with another physician. He may or may not suggest that you seek a second opinion regarding your breast cancer, but he will expect you to do that. Don't be intimidated, either, if the doctor questions the validity of a second opinion. It is your right and responsibility to search for another second opinion specialist, and any physician who questions that right should be removed from your list.

Dr. Petrek: Having a patient seek a second opinion is a routine occurrence for the physician, but very often women are embarrassed or reluctant to suggest it to their doctor.

Rebecca: I have encountered many women who were so comfortable with the surgeon who performed their biopsy and delivered the cancer diagnosis that they failed to research their second opinion options. Or they did go for an evaluation by another surgeon who did not analyze the case thoroughly and merely agreed with the first surgeon. Insurance companies report a very high confirmation rate on second opinions. Only a thorough search will give a woman the best possible chance of locating a quality specialist for her second opinion consultation.

I have interviewed many women who failed to obtain competent second opinions only to have years of uneasy thoughts that they may not have received the best care possible at the time. At a New York meeting of a breast cancer support group I met Sherry, a personnel consultant in her early forties. Most of us were currently in treatment and had had our surgeries within the past six months. Sherry seemed to have more than her share of problems. The surgeon had taken too much breast tissue during the lumpectomy to achieve a good cosmetic result, and her radiation marks were large and permanent and in obvious locations. She felt ashamed of her body and admitted that she should have taken more time for a second opinion by a qualified surgeon.

Dr. Petrek: It is important to see other specialists, especially those with practices not associated with the original surgeon. Very often doctors will recommend that a woman seek a second opinion from another doctor or colleague who practices with him at the same hospital. They act as each other's mutual referral service. If you can, try to see specialists in other towns or cities as well as those associated with different hospitals. The specialist is a doctor who has educational concentration and practices in a specific area of medicine. You would be looking for a surgeon whose patient base is largely women with breast disease.

Rebecca: You can begin your search for a breast surgeon specialist by asking for specific recommendations from your gynecologist, family physician, or friends, relatives, and business associates. Don't overlook the pharmacist, nurses, dentists, and other professionals that you know who work in health-related fields. You can call the breast cancer support groups in your area to get the names of regional breast surgeons and also the names of patients who might be helpful in assisting in your search for a specialist.

Because seeking a second opinion is an intelligent and effective support to a good medical diagnosis, many insurance companies and HMO's not only recommend but also require that their policyholders receive second opinions before they will authorize any surgery. Ask your insurance carrier or HMO if they have a list of breast specialists that they suggest you use in your area.

The largest hospital or medical center near you can also provide you with a list of breast specialists or, at the very least, could recommend a physician-referral service that you can call. Some hospitals have specific second-opinion referral services. Be wary, however, of services that are either run by physicians or those services that require payment by physicians for being listed.

Your state medical societies may also help you locate good doctors. You can use the Database in Part Five to locate facilities in your region. The national (1-800-ACS-2345) or state unit of the American Cancer Society, also listed in the Database, will give you a list of Cancer Centers with their telephone numbers to obtain a list of their breast surgeons. The National Cancer Institute in Bethesda, Maryland (1-800-4-CANCER), will also provide you with the names and addresses of qualified specialists in your area.

Dr. Petrek: As you gather your list of specialists you will want to examine where and how they direct their practice. For instance, are they involved in a multidisciplinary program or team approach to breast cancer treatment or are they physicians in private practice? There are advantages and disadvantages for the patient in both private and multiple-treatment approaches.

The multidisciplinary or team approach to breast cancer

diagnosis and treatment generally occurs at larger hospitals, medical centers, and cancer centers. It is a complete plan for treating breast cancer.

You probably will have already seen two or more physicians related to the diagnosis of your breast cancer and will be seeing many more before your treatment is completed. You may have seen your gynecologist and/or your family physician, a radiologist who examined you and your mammogram, and a surgeon who performed your biopsy. For the additional surgery that you may need you should be consulting with a breast surgeon specialist, and possibly a radiation oncologist if you choose lumpectomy, a medical oncologist if chemotherapy is suggested, rarely preoperatively but possibly after surgery, and a plastic surgeon if you think mastectomy with reconstructive surgery might be a better choice for you.

In larger medical complexes and cancer centers you will be under the care of several doctors at once, and they should be coordinating your treatment. At the time you meet with a breast surgeon specialist for your second or third opinion, you can also meet with other staff specialists to discuss the various treatment options available to you. All of these physicians will help you when it is time for you to reach a decision. These specialists are very often leaders in breast cancer research and treatment. They can practice their specialties with the latest in available research, specialty equipment, and expertise.

On your list of breast surgeon specialists you will find many who are in private practice. Some are highly experienced in the treatment of breast cancer, but many are not. Doctors can have very different educational backgrounds and experience. It doesn't matter that your doctor is highly regarded in the medical community if he or she is not experienced in treating breast cancer.

It is important to carefully research all physicians on your list who you will consider having to deliver your second or third opinion. Unfortunately, there is no board certification in breast surgery, or even cancer surgery, only in general surgery. This means that you are going to have to probe deeper into his practice to discover whether he is a breast surgeon specialist or just a surgeon who performs some breast surgeries.

Rebecca: You can check the doctor's credentials in the Directory of Medical Specialists or the American Medical Association Directory of Physicians. Both books can be found in your local library. You may also want to call the American Board of Medical Specialties (800-776-2378) to check that your doctor is certified. While board certification does not guarantee that you will have found a first-rate surgeon, you will at least know that the formal training and examination requirements have been completed. Ask another doctor, either a physician who has treated you in the past or a doctor or nurse who is a friend, for his or her opinion. You want to be confident that your surgeon is respected by his colleagues, has good judgment, will have genuine concern for your well-being and that he will listen and respond to your questions. To some women these qualities can be as important as good operating skills. You will have a long-standing relationship with this doctor, so select him or her carefully.

Many people who have breast cancer are treated by general surgeons who are not cancer specialists. This could result in treatment that is not state-of-the-art. In some cases the surgery is performed by the local physician and it is only when a recurrence is discovered that the patient is referred to a cancer center or large hospital experienced in cancer treatment.

By then, however, it may possibly be too late for a successful cure. While almost any competent general surgeon can perform a biopsy, he may only do a dozen or fewer mastectomies or lumpectomies in any given year. That is not many when you consider that many surgeons perform the operation several times per week.

The lumpectomy or mastectomy is not just a cut in the breast. It usually is accompanied by surgical removal of all or a portion of the lymph nodes in the armpit. This is a tricky piece of surgery that if not performed correctly can tend to predispose a condition known as lymphedema. Lymphedema is a swelling of the arm on the side of the lymph node surgery. I have seen many women with this problem and in some it is relatively minor but others can have large, bloated arms. This condition can be uncomfortable and temporary or can become a permanent problem. Lymphedema can occur at any time following breast cancer surgery, but usually in a small percent of women, approximately 2–4 percent, it is bothersome. Why take this risk when you do have other options.

Dr. Petrek: There are advantages as well as disadvantages in both the multidisciplinary approach and the private practice treatment. It can be difficult for a woman to decide which approaches are going to be best for her, depending on the stage of her disease and her personal lifestyle. Since the most common treatments for breast cancer are surgery, radiation, and chemotherapy, the majority of cancer specialists would probably agree that the team approach is the most complete.

If a breast cancer patient requires more than one treatment or an alternative therapy, such as surgery and radiation, or surgery and hormone treatment, or surgery, radiation and chemotherapy, the treatment plan should be administered by the respective specialists. At a large regional medical center, a university hospital, or a cancer center, you will often have several specialists with whom you can discuss a plan of treatment. You will have the advantage of the latest treatment and technology, which may not always be available at smaller medical institutions.

Rebecca: Yet the specialist or surgeon in private practice has great appeal for many women. They like the feeling of privacy and security in having a single doctor or a small group of doctors care for her. And many women seem to like the feeling of a personal doctor-patient relationship that a single practitioner offers.

It can be dangerous, however, to place your care in the hands of a single doctor. Cancer specialists usually recommend that patients submit to review by groups of doctors, not just a single doctor. We know that women typically may not disagree or argue with their doctors. They seem to be reluctant to speak up if they think there might be a problem. With many doctors watching over her breast cancer, a woman should feel secure that she is receiving the best possible treatment.

What very often happens is that a general surgeon, usually practicing at a local hospital, will perform the required surgery and schedule occasional follow-up visits. His breast surgical practice has increased over the years due to the high incidence of breast cancer.

Because he may have a varied surgical practice, however, he may not find the time to stay on top of recent developments in breast cancer treatment. A woman should ask herself whether a particular surgeon, even though his surgical skills are adequate, might not have a sufficient breast cancer practice to stay knowledgeable on the current forms of treatment. Or worse, she should ask herself if he can provide her with the appropriate therapy that would be best for her type of breast cancer. These are sophisticated questions that can be difficult for a woman to come to terms with, especially if she is comfortable with the current medical situation.

It is also appropriate to mention here that the general surgeon competes for patients with the breast surgeon specialist. He may not recommend that a patient go to another doctor if he feels he can do the same surgery. Unless the cancer has spread, the general surgeon may suggest that he take control of her surgery and schedule her follow-up care.

You, however, are the medical consumer, and you can and should shop around. Take your business to another doctor if you are not completely satisfied that this is the best doctor for you. Remember that the time delay of an additional week or two before treatment is really negligible in the time span of a cancer which may have started growing several years previously.

SPECIALIST CHECKLIST

1. Definitely seek one or more second opinions. You cannot make informed treatment decisions without them.
2. The quality of your second opinions is crucial to your receiving proper treatment. Approach the best specialists in the field of breast cancer both in and out of your regional area.
3. Vary your second opinions. For instance, see a private practitioner, a team of specialists, and another specialist at a major cancer center.
4. Check their credentials and their reputations. Ask their

office where they have hospital affiliations. Ask the hospitals how long they have been there. Are they involved in breast cancer research and clinical trials? If they are not they may not be up-to-date on the more recent surgeries or treatments.

5. When diagnosing and treating breast cancer, very often the best-quality treatment can usually be had at the larger hospitals with the latest equipment and the leading specialists. Larger facilities use modern treatments to produce their successes. You want to have one of them.

6. Remember, you call the shots because you are the consumer. Shop around carefully.

7. When you call to make an appointment, explain that you have a breast cancer diagnosis and are looking for another opinion. They will no doubt be able to give you an immediate (two to five days) appointment.

8. When scheduling your second and third opinion consultations, space them at least two or three days apart. That will allow the doctor time to review your mammogram, tissue slides, and pathology reports.

The Consultations—Meeting the Specialist

Rebecca: Your suspicions about breast cancer have been medically confirmed, and you have begun an all-out investigation to educate yourself so that you can make wise decisions about whom to see and where to go to be treated. You have a good sense by now about what options are available to you but you probably have many unanswered questions.

The best way to receive the most up-to-date information about the latest in treatment options is to communicate effectively with the physician specialist. The information that you provide them and the questions that you ask will give you more detailed information about your own personal breast cancer. The consultations will enable you to acquire additional information, provide you with another judgment on the medical diagnosis, and give you the opportunity to evaluate whether a good doctor-patient relationship can exist for the duration of your treatment. This will help you make a timely decision about how and by whom you will be treated.

By now you should have accumulated enough information about breast cancer to fill a file cabinet. The material should be organized so that it makes sense to you and will enable you to retrieve the information as needed. I had a master file of publications that I considered important for reference which I carried with me when making telephone calls and medical appointments. I found it helpful to keep separate manila file folders for:

Bills and other expenses
Insurance forms—blank, in process, and completed
    Medical and pathology reports
Test and scan results
Personal medical history
List of questions with supporting notes

You should have a large briefcase or heavy-duty file that will accommodate your:

Mammogram X rays
Tumor slides
Several copies of each of the written test or scan results, pathology, and medical reports
Several copies of your medical history
Several insurance forms already completed
Insurance and/or Medicare card
Hospital ID card
VISA, MasterCard, or American Express credit cards
Several blank checks
Microcassette recorder
A blank notebook
Master appointment calendar
Something distracting to do or read

This may be viewed as overorganization, but time is wasted if you have to reconstruct your medical history or fail to have the correct information when asked. This may well be the most stressful period for every woman in dealing with a breast cancer diagnosis. And when under stress we tend to be forgetful and disorganized. With your resources in place, you can confidently schedule the needed second opinion consultations.

From your priority list of specialists, call the top two or three for appointments. Some professionals will say that only one second opinion is needed. I disagree. Breast cancer diagnosis and treatment decisions are never made easily. And, we are dealing with *cancer*. I consulted with four specialists before making my decision, and I needed all four in order to feel completely satisfied with my decision.

Breast surgeons are in great demand and naturally booked but you will be surprised at how easy it is to schedule immediate appointments. Tell the nurse or receptionist that you have been recently diagnosed with breast cancer and would like to schedule a consultation.

Don't schedule two or three in the same day or even the next day. Leave one or two days in between because each doctor may want his own hospital or laboratory pathologist to review the tumor slides, and he may want his radiologist to read your mammogram X ray. This might take a day or two. If you live in a rural area and will be traveling to a major hospital, plan to stay overnight with friends or at a hotel if necessary.

Ask what medical information the doctor needs; the Cancer Worksheet in chapter 7 will help you formulate a complete medical history. Inquire as to what billing or insurance information they will require and make certain you have adequate directions to his office, clinic, or hospital. In some facilities you need a Ph.D. just to locate their offices. In short, it may take two months to see your dentist, but in two days you can see the best breast specialists. They recognize the urgency of your situation and will make every effort to be accommodating.

Prior to your consultation you will want to have formulated a list of questions that are of concern to you about your breast cancer. At the end of this chapter the consultation checklist includes some questions that you might typically ask the specialist.

At the same time that you are preparing a list of questions to ask the doctor, you will also want to think about what you consider necessary in a good doctor-patient relationship. For instance, you have spent a great deal of time studying breast cancer and preparing yourself for the consultations. Do you want a doctor who tells you that too much knowledge will frighten and confuse you, or do you want a doctor who respects the fact that you have made the effort to inform yourself and that you will be a cooperative participant in your own treatment? Do you need a doctor who will cater to your emotional needs and your psychological well-being, or is that less important than his being an excellent surgeon?

I felt that a superb cut was more important than a comforting bedside manner. However, another woman might need a sensitive, sympathetic, attentive specialist. Only you can evaluate and determine whether a particular physician will best meet your needs.

The second opinion consultations are for your benefit, and your evaluation of the specialist is just as important as his evaluation of your diagnosis. You should be alert to how he runs his office. For instance, does the doctor have adequate staff that is polite and helpful? Are you kept waiting for an inordinate length of time? Or were you rushed through the entire consultation? Does the doctor provide pamphlets, literature, and reading material on breast cancer? Are the facilities clean and up-to-date? For instance, does the examining room or office have a radiology view box with light for viewing mammography films? Are there needles, glass slides, and fixative solution for pathology preparation? If the facilities aren't up to date, he may not be either. You want to be wary of a doctor who is an expert in other fields. An obvious specialty in another area could indicate that the volume of breast surgeries he performs may not be great.

Does he sensitively respond to your concerns and does he answer your questions to your satisfaction? You want to be clear on his rationale for the diagnosis and treatment recommendations. In short, use your intellect when evaluating his medical expertise and your instincts when measuring the intangibles.

Prepare Yourself

Organize

Once the second opinion appointments have been scheduled you will need to organize the information you are going to deliver to the specialist. In brief you will need to have:

1. Copies of all tangible medical evidence of your breast cancer diagnosis; mammogram X ray, ultrasound report, tissue slides, pathology reports, test or scan results, surgical biopsy report, and any other pertinent medical information
2. Several copies of your medical history
3. Several insurance forms completed with the necessary personal information; your insurance and/or Medicare card; your hospital ID card
4. Blank checks and credit cards for payment
5. A file with your prepared list of questions and a notepad to record the doctor's answers
6. Your appointment calendar and a microcassette recorder

Plan Your Strategy

You will also want to plan a meeting strategy to make the consultation as productive as possible. You will want to:

1. Arrive on time and call if you will be delayed or need to reschedule the appointment
2. Be prepared to give the specialist the information on the tests and other medical results when he requests them
3. Have your list of questions and your notepad out of your briefcase and ready
4. Explain what you are hoping to gain from the consultation; try to engage in a dialogue in order to have your questions answered; don't try to impress the doctor with your knowledge on breast cancer—he will recognize this from the quality of your questions
5. Be prepared to answer questions concerning the medical history you have prepared; answer honestly and completely
6. Remember that you have asked for this consultation and you are looking for a second opinion—not necessarily the "easy out" to this diffficult diagnosis.

The examination by the breast specialist is like many other examinations you have already had by your gynecologist or family physician, and the surgeon who performed your biopsy. As women we view ourselves as modest and reserved when it comes to undressing. It became laughable when I thought about how many times I exposed myself to doctor after doctor. I felt like a flasher! Of course, the doctor was only concerned about the clinical aspects of my breasts, but I was surprised that after seeing so many doctors I rarely thought about disrobing.

This is the time when you will want your microcassette recorder handy. If the doctor allows it, and some will not, it is valuable in reconstructing the conversation and exchange of information. At any rate, have someone with you who can take good notes. Most physicians believe that good communication is an important element to good care.

CONSULTATION CHECKLIST

1. What is your evaluation of my medical exam and tests? The size of my tumor? The location? Do you suspect lymph node involvement? Do you believe that it has spread beyond the breast and lymph nodes? What stage am I in? What is my cure rate for that stage?
2. Do you concur with my original recommendation? If so, why? If not, why?
3. What is your surgical procedure? How much breast or breast tissue will you remove? Am I a good candidate for conservative surgery? Why? Why not?
4. What are your criteria for lumpectomy? If I choose lumpectomy, how much tissue will you remove surrounding the lump? Will that sacrifice a large portion of my breast? Do you evaluate margins?
5. What is your policy on lymph node surgery? Will you remove all lymph nodes, none, or a sampling?
6. Where will the scars be located? For the lumpectomy or mastectomy? For the lymph nodes?
7. Do you actually perform the surgery? Do you work with an assistant? How many breast surgeries do you perform in a month? Year? Do you perform more mastectomies or lumpectomies? (You must evaluate whether he is perfor-

ming enough breast surgeries to maintain breast surgical skills.)

8. At what hospitals do you have privileges? Do you work with a team of specialists? Do your colleagues look in on your patients? How available will you be prior to and after the surgery? Is there a tumor board for discussion of cancer cases? Will there be consultants on my case? Do you teach at a medical school? Do you do research on breast cancer? Do you have ongoing clinical trials, and can a patient participate?

9. Will you pass along a patient to a cancer hospital when treatment is beyond your control? Where do you suggest?

10. How much time do you think that I can safely wait for my surgery? Can you schedule me within that amount of time?

11. What are the specific risks to this particular surgery? What are the risks if I don't have it? Will you require additional tests?

12. What tests will be performed before the surgery?

13. How do you decide what postoperative treatment to recommend?

14. What is the length of my hospital stay? When will I be able to return to work?

15. What is the schedule for postoperative checkups during the first two years? Every three months? Six months?

16. Do you recommend psychological support following breast cancer surgery? Do you have a particular doctor that you recommend?

17. What can I do to get ready for my surgery? Should I avoid smoking? Alcohol? Are there any other drugs that I should avoid preoperatively? What can I do to assist in my recovery?

18. You could ask the secretary about the fees. Are they generally covered in full by insurers? Do insurers pay more for mastectomies or for lumpectomy and radiation?

CHAPTER 9

. . . .

Researching The Hospital

Rebecca: Most of us tend to think that the hospital in which we have our breast cancer surgery depends upon whom we chose to perform our surgery. In some instances this is true, but not always. Because breast cancer treatment can often require many visits to several doctors, as well as a variety of tests, you might want to consider for your second opinion a specialist who practices at a certain hospital. In general, good doctors have affiliations with good medical facilities.

There are many hospitals nationwide, ranging from the very basic to the highly sophisticated. Some hospitals are very large and specialized, while others are just large and provide a variety of services. Some hospitals are teaching institutions affiliated with large universities, and other hospitals are private or independent. Some hospitals have religious affiliations and are nonprofit, while others are profit-oriented.

If a hospital is not accredited by the Joint Commission on Accreditation of Healthcare Organizations, an organization endorsed by the American Medical Association, it may not qualify for insurance reimbursement. You will need to check with your personal medical insurer or HMO to verify that a hospital is acceptable for their coverage. It is important to differentiate among the various types of hospitals available for treating breast cancer and discuss the pros and cons of each.

Dr. Petrek: Why don't we begin with the 25 Comprehensive Cancer Centers in the U.S. In the Database in Part Five you will find a listing by region of institutions that have been recognized as Comprehensive Cancer Centers by the National

Cancer Institute. These cancer centers are subject to stringent and continuing review by the National Cancer Advisory Board.

This is where a woman might want to be for the complete treatment of breast cancer. There are a large number of specialists who concentrate on specific types of cancers. The patient receives a multidisciplinary diagnosis and treatment approach by on-staff medical experts.

Medical history is often made at these cancer hospitals. They initiate and participate in many research projects simultaneously, and they offer clinical trials and experimental treatments. They are often on the "cutting edge" in surgical procedures and can offer the latest in treatments.

If you have a large tumor with a suspicion that it has spread, this is a hospital you will want to consider. They have well-trained, board-certified specialists and an advanced level of technological sophistication. The multidiscipline or team consultation with several staff specialists, the surgeon, radiation oncologist, possibly the medical oncologist and plastic surgeon, the nurses and social workers, should give you an idea of the approach of the Comprehensive Cancer Center in treating breast cancer.

Rebecca: Many physicians have a definite bias against the cancer center, and many that I have met clearly told me that they would not recommend that a woman newly diagnosed with breast cancer seek a specialist surgeon practicing in a cancer hospital. It has been my experience that some doctors feel that a woman with breast cancer need not be subjected to seeing other patients with visible gross deformities from other types of cancer or to see small, balding children in wheelchairs wearing baseball caps.

Virtually every woman I spoke with who had been treated at a cancer hospital said she never felt that way. They found comfort in being at an institution where all the patients have cancer. They responded to the sensitive care and support of the staff, who have all been trained to deal with people with a potentially fatal disease. All had the sense that they and their chosen physicians were giving them the best, most up-to-date care available.

Dr. Petrek: Then there are the academic health centers or the university hospitals. The university hospitals are affiliated with or controlled by the eminent medical schools located around the United States. Some university hospitals are public and others are private. Because they provide internship and residency programs that train new doctors, they can draw the top physicians, academicians, and researchers and bring them in to staff the hospital. The university hospital can provide a range of high-quality care. These hospitals are up to date in the latest research, medical, and surgical techniques. In some urban areas the most prominent physicians and well-trained specialists in their fields practice in university hospitals. They are well-equipped to handle the breast cancer patient and can provide a large variety of treatment programs. More than 50-60 percent of patients with small, localized breast tumors were being treated with lumpectomies at academic health centers or university hospitals.

Rebecca: The university hospital is not for everyone, however. There are some inconveniences that you should be aware. Because the university hospital is a teaching hospital you may be subjected to examination by students and residents. Your complete medical history may be taken by three or four different people. This may be beneficial, however, if a forgotten but important detail is picked up. Some women are afraid that they might be involved in some type of experiment or clinical trial. This does not happen unless you wish to participate, and then you will be completely informed.

Also, because your doctor can be on the university faculty, teaching in his specialty as well as doing research, he may have other doctors covering for him and you may be cared for by his associates. If you cannot arrange a consultation at a Comprehensive Cancer Center this is a good place to explore for a second opinion. Usually a large university hospital can be found within reasonable distance of your home. You can call the Association of Academic Health Centers (202-265-9600) for those hospitals near you, and then you can begin searching for specialists within those hospitals.

Dr. Petrek: Then there is the large medical clinic. We have all heard the names of large clinics such as the Mayo Clinic, the Cleveland Clinic, the Lahey Clinic. One difference between these large clinics and most hospitals is that they have physicians on staff, unlike the large hospitals that allow doctors the professional privilege of admitting their own patients. There are multidiscipline group practices with doctors working together with you who can provide you with complete medical care for your breast cancer from diagnosis through treatment management. The large and well-known clinics offer a variety of diagnostic services, usually under one roof, to treat the breast cancer patient. The clinics also are committed to research and education, not only for breast cancer but for other diseases and medical problems.

Rebecca: Like the university hospital, you do see many specialists, and this is not like having a single doctor available to you. I am told that because the doctors are salaried and will get paid regardless of the number of patients they see, they spend a great deal of time with patients discussing their medical problems and concerns. If you live within range of a large medical clinic, it is definitely worth a call to have a consultation with their breast specialist. The clinics are in great demand and it can take time to schedule an appointment at several of the more popular clinics.

Dr. Petrek, what about the many specialty breast centers? This would seem to be the ideal place for a woman to have a complete breast diagnosis.

Dr. Petrek: There are many comprehensive breast centers around the United States and one could be located near you. They are often attached to the major cancer centers, or are affiliated with the larger hospitals or academic health centers, or they can operate independently. The purpose of a breast center is to provide a woman with a "one-stop" approach to any breast problems and can be especially useful in determining an effective breast cancer diagnosis.

The breast centers were designed to bring together a team of experts, such as radiologists, surgeons, pathologists, medical and radiation oncologists, plastic surgeons, psychiatrists, psychologists, and other supporting professionals, so that a woman can have a comprehensive opinion and recommendation in response to a specific breast problem.

In addition to the specialized personnel, the breast center can also provide other services. Very often they will have complete diagnostic capabilities such as the latest in breast imaging equipment, sophisticated pathology analysis, and the ability to perform specific biopsies. They also can provide radiation therapy and coordinate drug or hormone therapy.

The breast center often will have available to patients specific support services such as personal or family counseling, nutrition and genetic evaluations, and physical therapy after surgery. The underlying concept behind the breast center is to have all of the technology and personnel necessary to supply a woman with either an early diagnosis of breast cancer or a schedule for preventive breast maintenance.

Rebecca: I can see why the breast center would be an excellent place for a woman to search for a complete breast diagnosis. She would have the multidiscipline consultations and the diagnostic procedures all done in one location. However, the breast center should be researched as carefully as any other medical facility you are considering. You should receive a referral or recommendation from your doctor or a reputable medical colleague.

Dr. Petrek: Also remember that any facility and even any small office can call itself a "Breast Center." There are no minimum requirements to use this name. A breast center may not have more than the basic diagnostic capabilities and may have a group of doctors merely on call, not a cohesive team of specialists. A majority of their practical may not even be breast disease. You will want to know if the center is associated with an accredited hospital. Since state regulations and accreditation standards vary, the Joint Commission on Accreditation of Healthcare Organizations (708-916-5800) can confirm the accrediting organization.

All of a center's physicians and technicians should be board-certified in their specialties. You can call the state medical licensing board to determine if any complaints or charges have been made against a particular physician.

Many breast centers are located in larger cities and are not necessarily available to many women. Because they are in or near large urban areas their costs can be higher than other facilities. A comprehensive facility that has office space for its physicians and state-of-the-art equipment is going to be more expensive. Your insurer or HMO can give you cost estimates on the diagnostic and surgical procedures that they typically cover so that you can compare the costs.

Rebecca: Unless you live in or near a large city the local hospital may not provide the specialists and services necessary for complete treatment. You have to honestly and objectively evaluate the facilities and resources available in your community. This is definitely no easy task for two reasons: one, because you are emotionally tied to your community, usually the hospital in which you had your biopsy, and to the surgeon who performed your biopsy; and two, as a layperson you are not exactly sure where to go, whom to see, what to do, or what to ask. The easiest, most comfortable decision to make is not to have a consultation elsewhere and follow whatever surgery and treatment the original doctor recommends. It bothers me to see women fail to investigate other facilities but unfortunately all too many do.

Evaluating the local hospital facilities for breast cancer treatment should be an intellectual exercise. Unfortunately, for most women it tends to be an emotional exercise, if they do it at all. For instance, a town with a population of 10,000 can often have a hospital that services a region of 30,000 people and have good facilities for treating general medical problems. Most community hospitals have good staff surgeons, radiation therapists, oncologists, and usually adequate support personnel. And, with 1,208,000 new cancer cases this year alone, the local hospital has, out of necessity, organized oncology units to treat the increasing numbers of cancer patients. However, at community hospitals only approximately 25 percent of newly diagnosed breast cancer patients were offered lumpectomies over mastectomies.

A woman should be asking herself questions about what her doctor has recommended and what the local hospital can do to provide the specific care she may need. She should ask whether the surgical facilities are adequate for the type of surgery she needs. Is the laboratory or pathology department adequate to prepare and assess her tumor or lymph nodes? Does it need to be sent away to a distant laboratory?

If she needs chemotherapy or hormone therapy, can the doctor or oncologist design an appropriate schedule? Can the hospital lab give her the latest cancer testing on her blood? How many breast patients are they currently treating in their oncology unit?

If she needs radiation, does the hospital have the latest linear accelerator machines and technicians specifically trained on those machines, or will she need to go to another location? Is that the reason why the surgeon recommended a mastectomy instead of a lumpectomy? Are there other doctors that she should be seeing in connection with her breast cancer?

Are there other women patients who have breast cancer that she can talk with or is there a nurse or psychologist that can help with emotional recovery? If she has an axillary dissection, are there facilities for rehabilitation such as physical therapy? She will want to get moving as soon as possible after surgery.

In addition to herself, a woman should ask these questions of her doctor, a nurse or other medical professionals, a breast cancer support group, and other local breast cancer patients. The Database in Part Five offers state and regional listings for information and support. If a woman is objective and receives less than satisfactory answers to these questions from a variety of sources, the local hospital is probably not equipped to handle her breast cancer. She can call the Association of Community Cancer Centers (301-984-9496) and the National Rural Health Association (816-756-3140) and ask if they have information on her local hospital. Combination therapies are an important part of breast cancer treatment, and it is unusual for one physician or one small hospital to be sufficient. According to the American Cancer Society, survival rates for breast cancer are better than 93 percent when diagnosed early and properly treated at the initial diagnosis. Appropriate treatment should take precedence over convenience. Can you in good conscience gamble on anything less?

HOSPITAL CHECKLIST

1. Verify that the hospitals you investigate are accredited and acceptable to your insurer. Ask locally to see if they are financially sound. If necessary, call the Joint Commission on Accreditation of Healthcare Organizations (708-916-5800).

2. Does the hospital have a commitment to quality? What does the physical plant look like? Is it constantly upgrading its facilities? Are patient rooms and public areas pleasant? Are they clean?

3. Are the doctors practicing at the hospital all board-certified in their specialties? Are the staff and technical personnel appropriately accredited in their respective fields?

4. How many cancer patients is the hospital currently treating? Of those, how many are breast cancer patients? Is there a special floor or designated area for women having breast surgery? Is their a Tumor Board that meets regularly for discussions of cancer patient cases?

5. Are programs and support services available for dealing with the emotional and physical aspects of breast cancer? Are they led by psychiatric social workers and rehabilitation specialists?

6. Does the hospital appear to function efficiently? Can you reach the doctor by telephone? The ease in scheduling of tests and appointments should give you an idea. Have there been any recent problems that have been made public, either in the newspapers or on television?

7. Can the hospital laboratory perform the sophisticated bloodwork associated with cancer diagnosis and the latest in follow-up testing? Is the testing site organized? Is there appropriate protection against blood-related diseases? Do they send specimens and tumor tissue to other laboratories for analysis?

8. Is the business office effective and up to date? Will they give you estimates of costs? An itemized copy of your account? Are the admission and the financial papers orderly? Is there staff to assist you? Do they process

insurance forms promptly? Do they inform you of third-party services and reimbursements? Ask what they do to insure the privacy and confidentiality of information regarding your diagnosis and treatment.

9. Is there a patient recreation area that offers a library, arts and crafts, music, cards, games, and activities? Do they have a beauty shop? Are religious services available?

10. Investigate the breast center. Is it appropriately accredited? Aside from mammography, what additional imaging capabilities do they have? Do they have a team of doctors with whom you can consult? Are they all board-certified in their respective fields? What is their availability? Where do they perform their surgeries? Radiation? Oncology? Have their practices?

11. Do you have the sense that this is a place where you will be comfortable for 3–4 days? Do they have appropriate procedures in place for follow-up care?

CHAPTER 10

....

What Are the Options?

Rebecca: The uncertainty of the last few weeks, as you have submitted to several physical examinations, one or more diagnostic procedures, and one or more surgical procedures, has given way to a diagnosis. Now you know for certain. You have breast cancer.

I can remember leaving the hospital after having had the biopsy and walking down Lexington Avenue in New York in a daze with tears streaming down my cheeks. How can this be? What rotten luck? Why me? Clearly I was not in the statistical majority. Most tumors are revealed on mammogram. Mine was not. The majority of breast lumps are benign. Mine was not. What next? What does this mean? I had to take the time to compose myself, digest the information I had been given, and then begin to formulate a plan of action.

Staging Your Cancer

Dr. Petrek: Once the diagnosis of cancer is clear from the results of medical examination, the diagnostic procedures, a definitive biopsy, and pathological analysis, your cancer needs to be "staged." Staging is a categorization that doctors have for evaluating the extent of your breast cancer. The stages are classified as Stage O, which is the most curable, through Stage IV in which cancer has spread to other organs. Each stage is based on certain information about your tumor such as its size, its type, its composition, and its containment or its spread to a distant organ. Each stage will explain the level to which your disease has progressed. The staging process is an effective communication tool that doctors need to plan your treatment.

Breast cancer treatment varies from stage to stage, and you should know what stage you are in because while you are gathering information and getting second opinion consultations you will be asked whether you are Stage O, I, II, III, or IV. In some of your reports you might notice letter evaluation of your stage; this is the TNM classification system. The T stands for tumor, N for regional lymph nodes, and M for distant metastases. The letter T is assigned a number from 1 to 4 that will describe the size of your tumor or the level of invasion. X means not assessed, and O means no involvement. You cannot be completely staged until after lymph node surgery and the pathological evaluation of your nodes.

It is important for you to know the staging classifications with accompanying descriptions of what they mean. Following is a brief description of clinical staging:

STAGE O: A tumor that is confined to ducts or lobules. It is noninvasive or has not spread.
A total mastectomy without lymph node removal, or lumpectomy with or without radiation, can be the recommended treatments.

STAGE I: A tumor that is 2 centimeters or less in size. There is no evidence of distant metastases or spread to lymph nodes.
Lumpectomy and radiation or sometimes modified radical mastectomy might be the recommended treatment.

STAGE II: A tumor that is between 2 and 5 centimeters in size.
There is suspicion of lymph node involvement.
Modified radical mastectomy or lumpectomy with radiation may be recommended.

STAGE III: A tumor that is larger than 5 centimeters in size.
There is extensive breast involvement.
It may be rapidly invasive.
It has usually spread to the lymph nodes.
Preoperative chemotherapy might be recommended before a modified radical mastectomy or rarely a lumpectomy.

STAGE IV: A tumor of any size.
It has spread to other organs.
Immediate and long-term chemotherapy would be recommended.

You can see how important staging can be when designing a treatment program. In your reading you will often see statistical analysis relative to your particular stage. Keep in mind that the doctor treats you with the appropriate therapy that will be most successful, regardless of your stage.

Surgical Choices

Dr. Petrek: Not too long ago women had few choices when diagnosed with breast cancer. Up until as recently as twenty years ago the most common operation for breast cancer was a radical mastectomy that removed the breast, pectoral or chest muscles, and the lymph nodes. This operation is rarely performed now because studies have shown that this surgery is no more effective than the newer, less disfiguring modified radical mastectomy.

Today there are various surgical options available to women, and making decisions about them is not easy. Doctors, for example, could suggest one of two surgical treatments for early, less that 2 cm invasive breast cancer: a modified radical mastectomy, or a lumpectomy with radiation therapy. It will be your decision as to how you will proceed. You need to know what options you have and what treatment is available. You need that immediate, up-to-date information derived from your second opinion consultations. During the investigation you will have accumulated the resources needed to take a positive, proactive role in your treatment and health care.

Rebecca: Yes. Women have the right and the ability to decide for themselves what surgical procedure is appropriate for them regardless of whether the surgeon, husband, or family disapprove. It is your life and you can control what will happen to it.

Dr. Petrek: There are options when confronted with breast cancer today, but they depend most strongly on two issues: the composition of the tumor, and how far your breast cancer has progressed. Size of the tumor is important in that generally small tumors require less extensive surgery and usually less follow-up treatment. However, even small tumors can prove to be aggressive and send malignant cells to other parts of the body, either through the lymph nodes, or through the blood stream, or both.

Many combinations of surgery, radiation, chemotherapy, and hormone therapy are used in the treatment of breast cancer, and it can be confusing to be confronted with different opinions from different doctors practicing in different locations and under different circumstances. All do agree, however, that early detection is the key to minimal surgery, successful treatment, and cure.

"Lumpectomy" is a surgically conservative, breast-saving form of treatment for small breast tumors and is generally the obvious first choice if recommended to women. Rough estimates indicate that 50 percent of women diagnosed with breast cancer are candidates for lumpectomy. It is the surgical removal of just the malignant tumor with margins of surrounding normal breast tissue and lymph nodes in the underarm or axilla. The tumor with surrounding marginal tissue and the lymph nodes are sent for pathological analysis to evaluate whether they are free of cancer. The lumpectomy is almost always followed by radiation therapy, and in some cases chemotherapy. Breast radiation therapy after a lumpectomy takes six weeks, and treatment is five days a week.

Most breast cancer experts agree that for lumpectomy a team of specialists should be consulted. A surgeon, pathologist, radiation oncologist, and chemotherapist or medical oncologist can cooperate to plan the best possible treatment program. This means that you will probably have to go to a facility where this multidisciplinary treatment is available.

In the past this was controversial treatment for breast cancer at many hospitals, but currently it is the most popular form of surgery for small breast tumors. Doctors at large hospitals, medical centers, and major cancer centers consider lumpectomy to be just as safe as more extensive surgery. Conserving the breast is followed with radiation therapy and, in some instances, hormonal therapy or chemotherapy. The cosmetic results are excellent, the breast looks almost the same as it did prior to treatment, and it is worth the inconvenience of postsurgical radiation therapy. (Details of radiation therapy are covered in chapter 11 on follow-up treatment.)

With the arrival of lumpectomy as a comparable surgical choice, women with a suspected breast cancer no longer need to delay for fear that mastectomy is the only treatment.

However, not everyone is a good candidate for lumpectomy, even though it may be cosmetically preferable. The size of the breast, the location and size of the tumor, the type of incision, the effects of radiation on the skin, and the pathology of the tumor are all taken into consideration and will influence a decision whether or not to undergo a lumpectomy. Women whose tumors are too large or whose cancer is more extensive will not be good candidates. Also, women who have multiple cancers in one breast or whose cancer is attached to the pectoral muscles will probably need a mastectomy.

Rebecca: For instance, a woman in Phoenix called me at the request of a mutual friend. She was disturbed that her doctor had not recommended lumpectomy as a surgical option. The doctor had said that the tumor was just under the nipple and in a difficult location for breast-conserving surgery. She made peace with this diagnosis and is perfectly comfortable with her decision to have a mastectomy.

Dr. Petrek: Another surgical option for a woman with a breast cancer diagnosis is the modified radical mastectomy. Simply stated, this is the surgical removal of the breast and the underlying lymph nodes in the axilla or underarm. Nationally, this is still the most common surgical treatment for breast cancer. Over half of the women diagnosed with breast cancer are treated with mastectomies.

Even though conservative treatment is appropriate for some, there are many sensible reasons for a woman to choose a mastectomy over a lumpectomy. First and foremost, for many women the fear of cancer, a recurrence of cancer, or a strong family history of cancer makes the lumpectomy seem risky. Some women just aren't comfortable keeping a breast that they know contained cancer. They have a greater sense of well-being and peace of mind in knowing that the breast tissue has been eliminated by the mastectomy.

Secondly, some women are frightened by the thought of radiation therapy; and, they can't or won't commit to the time needed to complete the six weeks of necessary radiation treatment. Also, if they are geographically distant from a radiation therapy center they might choose to have a mastectomy.

Third, a woman who is pregnant and diagnosed with breast cancer would choose mastectomy rather than subject her unborn baby to radiation.

Fourth, for other women the tumor may be too large, or too extensive, possess microscopic factors to indicate a higher breast recurrence, or poorly positioned to consider any other form of surgery rather than a mastectomy.

Fifth, if there are multiple tumors in the breast a mastectomy would be indicated. The radiologist might spot many small microscopic calcifications or other cancers on a mammogram that might indicate mastectomy as the better choice.

Sixth, for some women the size of the breast can determine their decision for mastectomy. A lumpectomy on a small breast does not always produce cosmetically good results. In this case a mastectomy and breast reconstruction may be a better option.

Seventh, for those women who have had a lumpectomy and radiation and find themselves with a recurrence in the same breast, they must have a mastectomy.

There is a third option that is rarely recommended to certain women who are at high risk and that is the bilateral mastectomy. Surgically, it is the removal of both breasts. Some women who have a high incidence of breast cancer in their family are candidates for this procedure. This is elective surgery, however, and it is important to take time to consider this option.

In considering your surgical options you will also be asked whether you will be having reconstructive surgery. This is a decision that will need to be made prior to your surgery if you wish to have immediate reconstruction at the time of your mastectomy. Several procedures are available, and you should research them carefully. Some surgeons are comfortable discussing the procedure, and others will refer you to a plastic surgeon who specializes in breast reconstruction.

Also, some surgeons would like you to wait three months or so before having reconstructive surgery. If the procedure is to be done concurrently with the mastectomy you will have to coordinate and schedule this with the breast surgeon and the plastic surgeon. If you choose, you may wish to wait three months or longer before proceeding with reconstruction, and certainly after chemotherapy if that is recommended.

Rebecca: The surgical choices you make now regarding your breast cancer are highly personal, and your decision should be based on thorough investigation and research. It is your right as an intelligent woman to evaluate the surgical risks and begin mapping out a treatment plan for yourself. For instance, a Long Island woman that I had met in the hospital had both breasts removed. Robbie had always thought that her large breasts were her most attractive feature and when she was first diagnosed with breast cancer had a lumpectomy on one breast. Unfortunately, she had one lymph node that contained cancer cells. She had two small children and a family history of breast cancer. Before radiation, she decided to reevaluate her doctor's advice and have a bilateral mastectomy after chemotherapy and have both breasts reconstructed at the same time. Breast cancer is rarely simple, and decisions do not come easily. Much thought and soul searching are necessary for a satisfactory solution to a difficult and emotional problem.

Evaluating the Statistics

Rebecca: I feel that it is important to include some information on the value of statistics. Most articles on breast cancer include some statistical data. Very often in securing a diagnosis the medical professionals will mention statistics with regard to the treatment they are recommending to you. How valid is that statistical data and can you relate it to your own breast cancer diagnosis?

Many breast cancer patients were appalled when in March of 1994 they learned that the results of a breast cancer clinical trial were derived from partially inaccurate data. The results of that investigation, published in the *New England Journal of Medicine* in 1985, revealed that lumpectomy combined with radiation is as effective a treatment for early breast cancer as mastectomy.

The studies were compiled from 5,000 physicians practicing at 484 academic medical centers and community hospitals, coordinated at the University of Pittsburgh, and directed under the supervision of the National Cancer Institute. Doctors had for many years used the results of that clinical trial in making treatment recommendations to their patients. Women made treatment decisions based on this data in conjunction with their doctors' advice.

Other independent studies conducted since that initial 1985 clinical trial of the National Surgical Adjuvant Breast and Bowel Project have confirmed lumpectomy and radiation to be as effective as mastectomy in certain patients with early diagnoses of breast cancer. However, these studies make women question the quality of medical research and the outcomes of clinical trial studies. As a result, some breast cancer patients question the validity of their own treatment plans.

The medical establishment too became aware that the National Cancer Institutes (NCI), funded by the National Institutes of Health (NIH), had been less than diligent in monitoring medical studies. NCI will impose more stringent guidelines when such studies are done by institutions receiving federal grants for research. What about the regulation of other studies not under the government umbrella?

The Office of Research Integrity (ORI), which investigates scientific fraud, has also released its findings of procedural and statistical irregularities, which added to the depth of misconception. Hopefully, this disclosure can serve as a basis for improving the scientific standard in conducting clinical trials: establishing stringent administrative guidelines regarding data and its method of process for participating doctors and institutions; creating the appropriate supervisory mechanism for auditing clinical trials; and providing for a timely policy of delivering results to the public.

Large clinical investigations are important to determine the effectiveness of certain surgeries, drugs, and treatments for breast cancer. Very few medical advances would be made without them. As patients, however, we should question our doctor when asked to participate in a clinical trial. At the very least, we should know what the rationale, length of time, and objectives of the study are. What other medical institutions will be affiliated with the project? What therapies will be given in the course of the trial and how are patients selected to receive certain treatments? What is required of us as patients if we contribute our medical histories, our bodies, and in some cases our body tissue? How will our progress be supervised and by whom? And, how and by whom will the data be collected, formulated, analyzed, and ultimately be used?

I found it fascinating, frightening, and frustrating as I tried to gather specific information from many different sources. There were always the generic statistics that seem to be quoted in every article on breast cancer with little variation. But in other instances the percentage spreads on similar studies varied greatly from publication to publication. Much of the data was inconsistent and hard to evaluate, and there was a great deal of misinterpretation of the published statistics.

I recognize that specialized studies, with large numbers of patients enrolled, can produce diverse and sometimes contradictory results. Public trust in the quantity and validity of medical research, however, will most certainly be further eroded without some effort to consolidate the statistical information delivered to the public and to breast cancer patients.

Two troubling issues regarding the publication of statistical information surfaced as I sifted through articles on breast cancer. First, there was the length of time before results of clinical investigations were released in publications for the general public. To be a leading participant in a large medical investigation, involving some of the most distinguished academic health institutions, can bring national recognition and the right to publish the outcomes of the research. The conclusions of these studies are then submitted to journals for evaluation and subsequent publication. When the material eventually reaches the patient it has been summarized and rewritten in language that the general public can understand.

In almost all sources available to the layperson there is little mention of how the data was gathered, what research methods were utilized in the project, and what specific patient and treatment criteria were used by the study group to arrive at the conclusions. Without this specific information a woman diagnosed with breast cancer can hardly make an informed decision about her treatment.

And second, it can be months or years before those published research results are approved and are actually used by physicians in practice. Academic, medical, and governmental obstacles can create delays in bringing changes in surgeries, drugs, or treatments that doctors can safely recommend to their patients. Even when medical changes are approved for patient treatment, many doctors will wait before integrating the changes into their practices to determine the effectiveness of newer treatments.

It appears to be somewhat patronizing to those of us who have had lumpectomies within the last seven or eight years, to have independent studies rushed to publication supporting the conclusions of the flawed University of Pittsburgh investigation. We must live with our past treatment decisions, and those women with new breast cancer diagnoses must determine whether appropriate scientific study methods were employed before using the statistics as a basis for evaluating their own treatment options. It makes me wonder just how accurate those articles were in the publications that we read daily, weekly, and monthly.

The bottom line is that any statistical data on breast cancer is measured by definitive guidelines on selected women whose disease met very specific criteria. As much as we want answers, as patients we just don't have enough information about the specific cancers of the women who participated in the clinical trials to make comparisons about our own breast cancer. Therefore, it is important to be realistic when reviewing statistical data and not make premature evaluations about the information when relating it to our own breast cancers.

I prefer to think of breast cancer as an individual disease, not a group disease. Women defy the statistics and beat the odds every day.

CHAPTER CHECKLIST

1. Now you know. It is breast cancer. Have a good cry and then get tough. Develop a plan of action. Find up-to-date information. Call the cancer hotlines. Accumulate sources. Ask for help from the medical profession. The Database in Part Five will provide you with a list to get you started.

2. Go to your local library, a college library, and/or a medical library, and research your surgical options in detail. There is a wealth of information out there but you must spend time digging.

3. As you read, make notes, formulate questions, and prepare lists to ask the specialists with whom you will consult.

4. Learn as much about your personal case as possible. Know the composition of your tumor and the pathologist's interpretation of your report. Ask what stage you are likely to be in. Have your medical history up to date.

5. Keep an open mind. You have much information to absorb. Don't make a premature decision at this point.

6. Even the most reliable statistics may not apply to your case. Use the information selectively and wisely. Don't dwell on the negative data that may not have any bearing on your breast cancer.

CHAPTER 11

Follow-up Procedures

Rebecca: The fourth and final block of information necessary for you to make an intelligent treatment decision about
your breast cancer concerns the type of follow-up care you will
need after surgery. In May of 1988 the National Cancer
Institute (NCI) reported the preliminary, unpublished results
of three studies on breast cancer. In summary, it found that
women whose breast cancer had not spread to their lymph
nodes lived cancer-free longer after receiving both surgery
and chemotherapy or hormone therapy treatments. Those
women had their small recurrence rate cut by one-third to one-
half. NCI felt so strongly about these findings that it issued an
urgent "Clinical Alert" to 13,000 cancer specialists in the U.S.
recommending that adjuvant (additional) hormonal or chemotherapy could be significant to some women with Stage I breast
cancer. This means that many more women treated for breast
cancer today will have follow-up therapy of some type recommended to her.

If you think you will have a lumpectomy you will be given
radiation and possibly chemotherapy. If you choose to have a
mastectomy you might also want a breast reconstruction, or if
you need it, chemotherapy and/or radiation therapy. With
either lumpectomy or mastectomy, hormone therapy might
also be recommended to you. All of these treatment options
make the decision-making process complicated, and choosing
the course of treatment appropriate for you will depend on the
size of your tumor, on how far your cancer has progressed, the

pathology of your tumor, and what the risks are related to how much therapy you can or will tolerate.

Dr. Petrek: The decision you make regarding the type of surgery you have is directly related to the form of follow-up treatment you will need and vice versa. The decision on follow-up treatment must be made prior to your surgery. You will be presented with treatment recommendations that have been proven successful in the "cure" of breast cancer, and you will no doubt have questions. We can examine the options and alternatives available to you.

Radiation Therapy

The lumpectomy has become the preferred choice of breast surgery among American women today with early breast cancers, and breast radiation therapy is available at all cancer centers and most larger hospitals and clinics. The success of the lumpectomy, however, is dependent on the radiation therapy that follows surgery. In fact, physicians expect a commitment from the patient that she will follow the surgery with radiation therapy.

Radiation has suffered from bad publicity over the years, and the public perceives radiation as something to be feared. Women tend to think that radiation has been associated with some additional cancers, when in fact they should remember that it eliminates any residual disease in the breast. As mentioned in chapter 7 on risks, radiation causing breast cancer is a consideration in the youngest patients, such as those under the age of twenty-five.

In recent years, significant changes in radiation equipment have greatly improved the quality and safety of radiation treatment. Sophisticated radiation machines called linear accelerators have been added to cobalt machines and can produce more detailed and accurate fields in some breasts. The linear accelerator (LINAC) can deliver high-dose radiation to exact measured areas with little spillover that might affect the surrounding organs or tissue. Exact measurements are important, because you want the rays focused on the precise area to be irradiated, that is only the breast.

Radiation therapy decreases breast recurrences by delivering specific doses of energy directly to the breast, destroying any remaining cancer cells. The energy expended by machine is measured in units called "rads." A rad is the abbreviated term of measurement for "radiation absorbed dose" and is used when describing treatments using radiation. The radiation dose delivered to the breast is approximately 4,700–5,000 rads, 160–180 rads a day. You receive the treatment daily five days a week, for six weeks. The radiologist may suggest a boost dose of perhaps 1,000 rads directed at the primary tumor site, given over a period of a few days or weeks, depending on the dose.

Before you actually begin your radiation, you will be asked to report to the facility where you will be receiving your radiation therapy, usually within two to three weeks after surgery. This will not be for your first radiation treatment but will be a planning session with the radiotherapist and technicians.

The technicians use a simulator machine that operates like a linear accelerator or cobalt machine but does not deliver any radiation. A computer is used to precisely define the areas and angles to be radiated. The technicians usually prepare an upper body or breast mold to position and measure you so that each time you receive a treatment your body will be in the exact same location. Also, the technician will permanently, or semipermanently, mark specific spots on your body so that the radiation field is exactly the same each time. This simulation can take from one to three hours.

Rebecca: Radiation therapy is usually begun within four to six weeks after your initial surgery. This waiting period allows the body time to begin healing. Radiation therapy itself takes five or six weeks to complete, on a schedule of one treatment each day, five days a week, and is done on an outpatient basis.

I found it useful to schedule radiation treatments early in the day. In that way you can avoid the inevitable patient buildup that seems to occur at some facilities. Also, if a machine is under repair, being tested, or otherwise out of commission, you are in a good position to reschedule the appointment. You cannot miss an appointment without making it up. You are required to have the total planned dose of radiation therapy.

Dr. Petrek, are there any side effects that we should be aware of or precautions during treatment?

Dr. Petrek: There are very few side effects associated with radiation therapy. There is no pain, or nausea, or sickness. During the last week or two of treatment you may experience some mild fatigue. Some women experience temporary redness in the irradiated area, more like a mild sunburn or suntan. This is due in part to the expansion of the small blood vessels, in this case caused by the radiation from the rays of the machine and not from the rays of the sun. Your irradiated breast will probably be more firm with the passage of time, compared with your other breast, and possibly slightly larger. In general though, the appearance of the breast looks much the same as the nonradiated breast.

You may have a routine blood test taken periodically during treatment to make certain that the radiation is not causing your blood count to drop. You also will not be allowed to use underarm deodorants, perfumes, or powders to the chest and breast area, or body soaps that may contain aluminum or other metal that can interfere with the radiation.

Rebecca: The inability to use deodorants was a real problem for me. The cornstarch that the radiation oncologist suggested was inadequate. I did find a natural crystal deodorant that was much more effective. Another breast cancer patient had suggested that I use fresh aloe from the leaf of the plant during treatment. Following each treatment I broke apart a leaf and spread the gel on my radiated breast. I experienced only very minor redness to the skin. The side effects of radiation therapy appear small related to the beneficial effects. Radiation successfully eradicates cancer cells.

RADIATION CHECKLIST

1. You will need follow-up care in one form or another because those treatments significantly reduce recurrences;

ask your doctor what is recommended for you. How long will they take? What are the risks and possible side effects?

2. With radiation therapy, will the markings be permanent or temporary? Will an upper body mold be made? Will there be a simulation of the radiation process prior to actual treatment?

3. Do you have a choice of facilities? How many machines do they have? How many patients? Will the scheduling fit into your daily routine? Is there usually a long wait for treatment? Can you see the facility beforehand? Can you meet the technicians who will actually be giving you treatments? By familiarizing yourself with the facility and treatment areas, the procedure will seem less intimidating, and you will a have better indication about the timing of your treatments.

4. When and how often will you meet with the actual radiation oncologist to monitor your treatment? Weekly during treatment? Are there any postradiation symptoms or side effects that you should be looking for?

Chemotherapy

Dr. Petrek: Chemotherapy has long been in use to control cases where breast cancer has spread to distant sites in the body (metastatic cancer). With the May 18, 1988 Clinical Alert from the National Cancer Institute (NCI), however, more women with nonmetastatic breast cancer are given a chemotherapy program than ever before. The lymph-node surgery and the pathology of the lymph nodes help determine whether a patient would benefit from adjuvant chemotherapy. "Adjuvant therapy" is a limited series of chemotherapy treatments given in addition to the primary surgery or surgery and radiation treatments.

Since the NCI announced the results of three new breast cancer studies, chemotherapy or hormonal therapy has been recommended and given to many women with early breast cancer that has not spread to the lymph nodes. Never was a Clinical Alert met with such controversy among oncologists and surgeons. The medical profession could not agree on which node-negative breast cancer patients were at high enough risk for a recurrence and therefore would benefit from the chemotherapy.

Now, after more than five years, adjuvant chemotherapy is routinely started at the time of initial surgery in selected women with negative lymph-node status. This could mean that your doctor might well recommend adjuvant chemotherapy as follow-up treatment for your breast cancer.

Chemotherapy is the administration of a combination of chemical agents distributed throughout the body by way of injection into the bloodstream to attack and destroy the fast-growing cancer cells that have spread. Simply stated, the anticancer drugs circulate throughout your body to reach undetected cancer cells that may be there but are too few to be detected by the usual methods of X rays, scans, or blood tests.

The most common chemotheraputic drugs used in breast cancer treatment are cyclophosphamide (Cytoxan), methotrexate, 5-fluorouracil (5-FU), doxorubicin (Adriamycin), vincristine (Oncovin), and prednisone. Because each drug acts differently in attacking cancer cells these drugs are most successfully used together in combinations of two or more such as CMF (cytoxan, methotrexate, and 5-FU) or CAF (cytoxan, adriamycin, and 5-FU).

These drugs are delivered in measured doses in a variety of treatment schedules designed by your doctors. Cytoxan may be taken orally daily for two weeks a month, others may be injected once every three weeks and yet others may be injected once a week for two weeks a month for a minimum of six months. Chemotherapy treatments can be given in a doctor's office, clinic, or hospital under the supervision of an oncologist. Each oncologist has certain protocols that he uses depending on the stage of your cancer, the progression of your disease, and the condition of your general health.

Rebecca: I don't know of any form of medical treatment that brings out greater fear from people than the prospect of having chemotherapy. I can remember intellectually accepting the fact that I would undergo six months of adjuvant chemotherapy. However, I suffered a panic attack minutes before receiving my first chemotherapy treatment. Considering that the treatment was all over in less than ten minutes I wondered why I had been so anxious.

I think that chemotherapy is viewed as the ultimate treatment of last resort in a patient with cancer. While this is true in some cancers and even in extensive breast cancers, it is not always the case. Historically, women with breast cancer were not treated with chemotherapy until the cancer had metastasized throughout the body. Today, however, chemotherapy is suggested for certain Stage I node-negative women as a precaution against undetected spread of cancer.

Studies have clearly indicated that appropriate breast cancer patients treated with chemotherapy have lower recurrence rates, by one-third to one-half, and higher long-term survival rates. Personally, the survival numbers were such that I felt that I could put up with anything for six months and it was definitely to my advantage to have chemotherapy.

Dr. Petrek: The potential side effects of chemotherapy treatments are well documented and often unrealistically presented. Perhaps this is the major reason why some women who should have chemotherapy refuse to do so. Remember, the side effects can be different with each woman, and your reaction may vary depending on the combination of drugs your oncologist has recommended.

As in most cancer treatments, modern research has refined the use of chemotheraputic agents so that the same or better results can be obtained compared to drugs of the past which cause more side effects. The side effects are almost always temporary and will disappear once your treatment is completed. Moreover, most side effects can be minimized with counteractive drugs and in some cases can be prevented altogether.

Rebecca: The most traumatic side effect that women mention most often is hair loss. While some women do lose their hair, others experience only a slight thinning or very little hair loss. Hair loss is a temporary condition and in some cases begins growing back during treatment. For most women hair grows back thicker and healthier after chemotherapy is finished.

I lost all of my hair during chemotherapy treatment and it has returned exactly as it was before the treatments. During that period of roughly five months I accumulated a variety of wigs for specific occasions and activities, a collection of fabulous hats, and the most beautiful scarves I could find. Unless one knew me personally no one suspected that I was bald. I won't say there weren't times that I felt self-conscious and awkward, because there were. However, it became a challenge to try to be as creative and chic looking as possible.

Another side effect that concerns women is the nausea associated with chemotherapy treatments. Most women do experience some nausea while on chemotherapy, but it is a temporary condition and is treatable by drugs. At the time I was to have my treatment the nurse gave me a shot of Compazine to control any nauseous feeling that I might have within the first few hours after receiving the treatment.

The degree of nausea can be determined by the combination of drugs that your doctor recommends for you. Some cancers require specific chemotheraputic agents that make you more nauseous than others. Depending on the drugs you are taking most women do not experience anything more serious than mild nausea and general discomfort which decreases between treatments.

Some stomach problems and nausea can be controlled by a change in eating habits. For example, some women find that avoiding fat or fried foods or eating smaller meals more often can help with nausea. Salty and dry foods, such as crackers or toast, can help if you have been vomiting. Liquids and soft foods such as soups, juices, gelatin, eggs, and pastas can soothe the lining of the mouth and throat.

Dr. Petrek: The most serious problem patients can encounter while taking chemotherapy affects the white blood cells. With many programs, patients have a complete blood count (CBC) every week to monitor the blood elements to detect any changes or body reactions while on chemotherapy. This is usually by a simple finger stick and not by drawing blood from the vein. Bone marrow contains tissue that produces our red and white blood cells as well as platelets. The chemotheraputic agents suppress the bone marrow's production of white blood cells, leaving the patient with an abnormally low white blood cell count. White blood cells protect us from infection and when the white blood cell count drops below a certain level, treatment must be suspended temporarily to allow the bone marrow to produce more white cells. Platelets help make our blood clot and a low platelet count could lead to bleeding.

During this period most women feel tired and the body is susceptible to infection. Patients must take preventive measures to avoid illness. If this happens get additional rest. Ask your doctor about dietary guidelines to keep your body at its peak. The doctor may recommend increasing protein and calories, eating several meals a day instead of three large meals, taking nutritional supplements, and reducing alcohol intake. Also, you should ask which medications are acceptable for you to take while you are on chemotherapy.

Rebecca: Another side effect of chemotherapy in many premenopausal women is the interruption of their monthly periods. In some women, periods return to normal upon discontinuing treatment, while others remain in the menopausal state. This means that, in addition to not having a period, you will also experience some of the classic symptoms of menopause such as hot flashes or night sweats.

Chemotherapy treatments can cause oral complications in some women such as inflammation of the mouth, throat sores, gum disease, and accelerated tooth decay. While I never had a problem with these side effects I have known women who have had oral discomfort. As a precaution it is wise to see your dentist prior to chemotherapy for any dental work such as cleaning, filling cavities, and application of fluoride to help reduce any possible complications.

While you are on chemotherapy, sign on with a LOOK GOOD...FEEL BETTER "Caring For Yourself Inside and Out" program. This is a program created in partnership with the American Cancer Society, the Cosmetic, Toiletry, and Fragrance Association Foundation and the National Cosmetology Association. There are ACS units around the U.S. sponsoring seminars to help women who are on radiation and chemotherapy look and feel their best. Women are taught about makeup and hair and wig styling techniques to improve their appearance and self-image during treatments. Call 1-800-558-5005 for information in your area.

Hormone Therapy

Dr. Petrek: Hormone therapy is the most common form of follow-up treatment for women who have had breast cancer. Approximately 60 percent of breast cancer patients each year take hormone therapy following their surgery. Estrogen, the female sex hormone, was instrumental in the growth of our uterus, vagina, Fallopian tubes, and breasts at puberty, and our ovaries continue to manufacture it until we reach menopause, around the age of fifty. It has been known for some time that some breast cancers rely on estrogen for growth, and the Estrogen Receptor and Progesterone Receptor tests performed on your tumor at the time of the biopsy can determine this. If your ERA and PRA tests are positive, meaning that your tumor grows with the help of female hormones, you may be a good candidate for hormone therapy. A large percentage of the women who will be diagnosed with breast cancer this year will be placed on hormone therapy.

Prior to the discovery of estrogen-depressing medications, a woman's ovaries would often be surgically removed to curtail the production of that hormone. In fact, this was one of the first known treatments for breast cancer. Today, however, there is a drug called Nolvadex or tamoxifen that can be administered instead to block the estrogen receptors. Tamoxifen, taken in pill form and begun soon after primary surgery, has improved a woman's chance of long-term survival. The five-year studies indicate that appropriate women taking tamoxifen have a 38 percent chance of living longer without recurrence than women who do not take the drug.

In the past, hormone manipulation has proved most successful in postmenopausal women. Premenopausal women may also benefit from this treatment. If you were menstruating prior to your surgery but did not during chemotherapy your doctor might prescribe tamoxifen.

Rebecca: The use of tamoxifen in the treatment of breast cancer is one of the most important advances in recent years.

We know that while the estrogen in our bodies can promote cancers of the breast and endometrium (or cancer of the uterine lining), it does protect us against heart disease and osteoporosis. Tamoxifen is not without side effects, however. Without estrogen in our bodies we will experience the classic menopausal symptoms: dry and thin vaginal tissue; hot flashes and night sweats; sleep disturbances; urinary problems; psychological problems such as anxiety, depression, irritability, and concentration; infertility; and atrophy of the reproductive organs. Many of these symptoms can be managed through lifestyle changes such as a well-balanced diet rich in calcium to counteract osteoporosis, regular exercise to maintain bone density, reducing the stimulants in caffeine and alcohol, stopping smoking, and taking a daily vitamin supplement. These changes will not only promote a healthy body but ease the discomfort of menopause and postmenopause.

There are trade-offs that we must consider when evaluating whether to subject ourselves to hormone therapy that may last for a period of a few years to a lifetime. One thing that studies do not show and the doctors cannot tell us are the long-term effects of tamoxifen on our bodies.

While I was at the hospital having a routine checkup I asked about the tamoxifen studies. Specifically, I had wanted to know how long I would remain on the drug. While five or more years is typical, a curious situation is developing. Women are refusing to go off the drug in spite of their doctor's recommendations that they do so. What are we to do? This is yet another area where we are in a position of having to make decisions in determining our own medical treatment.

Dr. Petrek: A woman must balance the actual risks associated with a recurrence or metastasis of her breast cancer and the possible risks that might be associated with long-term tamoxifen treatment. The future risks are possible cancers of the uterus, ovaries, and liver. Studies are just now appearing that indicate women taking tamoxifen have a two to three times greater risk of developing uterine cancer than the general population. It also may promote growths of ovarian cysts as well as other types of tumors. In addition to reducing the possibility of a recurrence of breast cancer, however, tamoxifen does have the benefits of offering women some protection against osteoporosis and heart disease. A woman needs to consult with those oncologists administering the tamoxifen clinical trials to evaluate her own individual risks.

HORMONE THERAPY AND CHEMOTHERAPY CHECKLIST

1. Ask the medical oncologist what is recommended for follow-up therapy? Are they in favor of adjuvant chemotherapy? How aggressive? Hormone therapy?
2. If your doctor recommends hormone therapy ask him why he thinks it is necessary. What were the results of the estrogen and progesterone receptor tests? Will the drug be tamoxifen? Will it be combined with any other medication? What are the side effects? Should both chemotherapy and hormone therapy be given?
3. What will the hormone therapy do to my periods? Will this affect my ability to have children? Will I experience menopausal symptoms? What are the side effects?
4. If the doctor recommends chemotherapy, what is the reason for recommending that form of treatment? How long will you be in treatment? When will you begin? What drug combinations will be used? How will they work on your cancer? What are the benefits of such treatment?
5. What are the side effects of the treatment? How long will they last? Will medicines alleviate them? Are there any dietary restrictions, and should you see a dietitian? What other medicines might interfere with the chemotheraputic drugs?
6. What is the treatment schedule? How often will you have checkups while in treatment? Will the doctor see you prior to your treatment? Who will oversee the weekly blood work needed during treatment and advise you about the results?
7. Where will the treatments be administered? Is there an outpatient facility closer to home that can deliver the correct dosages? How are they given? How long will they take? Who actually will give me the drugs?
8. What services are available for help with my insurance,

financial aid, transportation, support groups, and other problems that might be associated with treatment?
9. What are the emotional side effects? Is there someone available that I can talk to if I experience anxiety or depression? Are any meditation or visualization techniques suggested?

Breast Reconstruction

Dr. Petrek: Another area for follow-up after breast cancer surgery is breast reconstruction. Breast reconstruction is the creation of a new breast to replace the one that has been removed by mastectomy. It is a surgical procedure that is available to many women at the time of their mastectomy, or within a few months of their mastectomy, or even many years after their mastectomy. If you are considering breast reconstruction, you should discuss this procedure with the surgeon prior to your breast surgery. The location of the mastectomy incision and the extent of the remaining skin may be important to the reconstruction procedure.

In addition, you may want to consult with one or more plastic surgeons prior to your breast cancer surgery to coordinate a plan for reconstruction that is appropriate for both surgeons. Many breast surgeons work with plastic surgeons when patients choose to have reconstruction on one or both breasts. Research the credentials of the plastic surgeon as carefully as you did for the breast surgeon using the information in Part Three as a guide.

Several procedures are most often used in reconstructing the breast, and you and your doctors will decide which technique is best following your breast cancer surgery. The timing of the surgical procedure is largely dependent on the follow-up treatment you require. For instance, if you will be having adjuvant chemotherapy your doctor might recommend that you wait on the reconstruction until after you have finished treatment. The choice of the type of surgical reconstruction is dependent on your breast size, your muscle tone, the condition of your skin, and on the state of your general health.

Rebecca: The reasons why some women choose to have

reconstructive surgery are individual. For some women it allows them to regain their self-confidence and self-esteem. Breast reconstruction makes them look good and feel better by cosmetically returning their body to its precancer appearance. It can offer women the chance to regain their feminine identity.

For many athletic women breast reconstruction offers them the freedom to compete without the nuisance of dealing with a prosthesis. Pat, a friend in Chicago who had reconstructive surgery, felt breast reconstruction was well worth the additional effort. She feels whole again, and, like most women who have new breasts, is willing to discuss the surgery with women who are considering breast reconstruction. I have friends who will "show and tell" if a woman is concerned about the surgical outcome.

Other women, however, are perfectly comfortable with their new postsurgical image and choose not to subject themselves to additional surgery. They also may have concerns about the future risks and complications associated with reconstructive surgery.

This is a personal choice that women give a great deal of thought and care to. While you need not make this decision immediately, you will want the surgeon to perform your breast surgery with the option of breast reconstruction at a later date.

Dr. Petrek: Briefly, let's examine the procedures available to reconstruct the breast.

The implant. This procedure involves the insertion of a pouch about the size of your other breast, filled with silicone gel or saline solution that is placed under the skin and chest muscle. The incision can be made in the mastectomy scar area or on the side near the armpit where there is enough skin and muscle to cover the implant. There may or may not be a drain inserted to alleviate any fluid that may accumulate.

This procedure can be performed in a fully equipped operating room in a doctor's office or in a hospital under general anesthesia. The procedure takes from 1 to 2 hours and costs range from $4,000 to $6,000. Insurance usually covers the cost of reconstructive surgery for medical reasons.

The expander-implant. This is the most common form of

breast reconstruction procedure. The expander is an elasticized pouch that can be placed in the breast either at the time of the mastectomy or subsequent to the mastectomy. The surgeon makes the incision in the mastectomy scar and inserts a deflated expander under the skin and muscle. Once it is in place the surgeon then injects a small amount of sterile fluid into the expander.

Each week for a period of 8 to 12 weeks you will visit the surgeon for additional injections of fluid to gradually enlarge the expander to the approximate size of the other breast. When the appropriate size has been reached, the surgeon then removes the expander and inserts a permanent implant.

The initial operation for insertion of the expander can be done at the time of the mastectomy or later under general anesthesia. The surgery takes 1 to 1½ hours. The implant procedure can be done as an outpatient in a doctor's office or hospital under local anesthesia. The cost for this type of reconstruction ranges from $5,000 to $7,000.

The tissue transfer. This surgical procedure is infinitely more complicated than the implant or expander techniques in that it involves the movement of tissue from other parts of the body to the breast area. Muscle tissue is usually used from the abdominal or "rectus abdominus" area and rarely from the back near the shoulder blade, called the "latissimus dorsi" area. In both cases body tissue is moved under the skin from the back or abdominal areas to the chest area and molded into the form of a breast. Additional incisions depend on which procedure is selected. Both procedures rarely may require additional implants to add to the muscle tissue to produce a breast of the appropriate size. The surgical procedure is lengthy, around 6 hours, and requires 6 or 7 days in the hospital. The cost is $7,000 to $15,000.

Regardless of the reconstructive procedure, either the implant method or tissue transfer method, most doctors will recommend that you wait a reasonable period of time before making the nipple and areola. The reason for the wait is so that the breast has an opportunity to settle into its location and any shape or position readjustments can be made when the nipple and areola are made. When the nipple and areola are reconstructed, tissue can be used from the other nipple, the upper inner thigh, behind the ear, or the vaginal lips. This surgery takes from 1 to 2 hours and costs $2,000 to $5,000.

Rebecca: This is a brief overview and should give you a base from which to research which procedure may be best for you. There are several good books and pamphlets available on breast reconstruction, and you should read in depth about the specific procedures you might be considering before you make a decision.

In considering breast reconstruction you should research the specialists and hospitals. Prepare for your consultations with the plastic surgeons in the same manner as preparing for the consultations with breast surgeons that was discussed in chapter 8.

Effective communication with the plastic surgeon involves asking questions about the type of surgery that may be appropriate for you. As with all surgery, there are risks and complications that will have to be reviewed with the plastic surgeon. You want a plan of action formulated before you have your initial surgery for treatment of your breast cancer and you want your doctors not only surgically coordinated but in agreement about what is appropriate for your type of breast cancer. While you may not always know what type of operation you should have at the outset, by researching a plan of action you will leave yourself open to future surgical options.

RECONSTRUCTION CHECKLIST

1. You would like to explore the possibility of reconstruction. Does your doctor recommend that it be done at the time of mastectomy or at a later date? Why?
2. Is there a plastic surgeon that is recommended? How many reconstructions do they do together? What is the most common procedure that they do? In what hospital?
3. What type of reconstructive procedure does the plastic surgeon recommend for my type of breast cancer? What is the surgical procedure? Will there be additional scars or will the plastic surgeon use the mastectomy scar?
4. What type of implant is used? Have there been any com-

plications with the implant? How does it look and feel under the skin? Will the plastic surgeon be able to match my other breast?

5. What is the recovery period? For implant surgery? For tissue transfer surgeries? Will the plastic surgeon show you photographs of other patients who have had the procedure you are considering done? What about names so that you can speak with them?

6. What is the surgical technique preferred for reconstructing the nipple? How long must you wait before the procedure can be done? How long does it take? Where is it done? Are there any risks involved?

Postsurgical Care

Rebecca: When a woman has and is treated for breast cancer, she becomes a changed person from that time on for the rest of her life. She knows that she is different. She begins a lifetime of annual mammography, the monthly practice of breast self-examination, and she watches for possible recurrences of cancer in and around her breasts. She is also looking for symptoms that might indicate cancer at other locations in her body. In your consultations you will want to know your doctor will be available to you in the years that follow your breast cancer. If that is not the case, and academic doctors in particular can change locations, then there should be a colleague or an extensive hospital support system that can watch you medically.

Dr. Petrek: The timing of your doctor's follow-up care can depend on the type of surgery you have had and what treatment you had following the surgery. For instance, if you had a lumpectomy followed by radiation therapy and chemotherapy you would see the breast surgeon and the radiation oncologist for a breast/chest exam every 3 or 4 months for 2 to 3 years. The medical oncologist is an internist and has his own schedule depending on the internal medicine aspects of the breast cancer. You would be on alternating schedules for the three doctors thereafter.

Of course, if there are complications you would seek

additional treatment. Lymphedema is a common condition which can affect breast cancer patients. As discussed in chapter 8, this is a buildup of lymphatic fluid causing a swelling in the arm on the side where you had your lymph nodes removed. This occurs in approximately 2 to 4 percent of breast cancer patients. Because the pathology of your lymph nodes is critical to your treatment, the surgeon must remove some or all of them as well as cutting the vessels that connect them. Lymphedema is a condition treatable either by your breast surgeon or a rehabilitation specialist that has experience with the condition. There are exercises you can do that will stimulate the lymph circulation. Elevating the arm periodically can also help. You can wear an elastic sleeve that compresses the arm and hand, and, if serious, a daily mechanized compression of the arm can be administered to remove the accumulated fluid.

Rebecca: A portion of your lymph nodes have been removed and even though other lymph nodes in your body take over to make up for that loss, you will have to take care to protect the affected arm from infection. You will want to question the doctor as to what precautions he or she feels are necessary after surgery to guard against infection. The doctor probably will suggest that you keep from getting any cuts, scratches, bites, or burns on the arm. It is better if you don't wear any tight, restrictive clothing or jewelry on your arm, or carry heavy bags or suitcases with the affected arm. You should call immediately if your arm becomes swollen, hot, or red. Ask what you should do if this occurs.

At the same time you are watching your physical health for signs of recurrence, you should be aware of your mental well-being. Studies have shown that many women become temporarily depressed following breast cancer surgery and can experience low periods for some time after treatment. Depression can naturally follow a diagnosis and treatment for cancer but, depending upon the circumstances, women who have undergone reconstructive breast surgery seem to suffer less emotional distress than those who have not had reconstruction following mastectomy. Women who have been treated with the lumpectomy and radiation procedure seem to recover their emotional equilibrium much more quickly than those who have mastectomies.

I made an interesting discovery at a lecture on breast cancer at the American Cancer Society in New York recently. A psychologist who treats depression in breast cancer patients stated that women who have had lumpectomies suffer from not having their cancers taken seriously by their families and friends because of the breast-conserving surgery they have had. Ask your doctor what is available in your area for follow-up psychological counseling either by a psychiatrist or a hospital social worker. It is definitely helpful to know that you have someone on whom you can call during periods of anxiety and depression.

Any surgical procedure for cancer and its follow-up therapy can prove traumatic. You may experience emotional imbalances or disturbances because of the hormone therapy or chemotherapy you are taking, especially in the beginning months. In addition, the radiation schedule may cause stressful time constraints. Then, when all treatments have ended, you may feel anxious and worried that you are no longer taking any positive action to help yourself. This too can be stressful and psychologically unsettling, as you try to strike a balance in your life between your history of cancer and a future faced with fear and watchfulness for recurrence.

Your emotional well-being following cancer is directly tied to your confidence that you were appropriately and successfully treated. I found that women who did not take the time to research the specialists and their hospitals or have the second opinion consultations, spend years questioning whether they had adequate surgery or received appropriate treatment for their breast cancer. The reward of thorough research is peace of mind for your future. That is not to say that your cancer won't come back. It might. However, it will not recur because you failed to take positive action during the diagnosis. And it won't happen again because there was better treatment elsewhere and you didn't take the time to locate it. It is your life that is important here, and you are the only one who can take responsibility for the choices and decisions that will affect your future.

POSTSURGICAL CHECKLIST

1. What does your doctor recommend for follow-up care? How often will you need your checkups? What tests, scans, or X rays are required? How often?
2. If you have been treated by a team of specialists, how do they determine the schedule of who sees you and when so that you avoid duplicate trips to the hospital for tests? How do they confer? Are reports sent to each of them independently or to a master file? Whom do you call for medical advice?
3. What should you do if you develop lymphedema? How many of your doctor's patients develop this condition? What treatment does the doctor usually recommend to correct the problem? What does this condition mean for you medically in the long run?
4. What can you do when you need psychological assistance? Are there support groups at the hospital or community organizations? Do special patients with similar conditions exist that you can speak with?
5. Fight that reticent attitude that we all have that prevents us from asking the important questions. You need information, and the professionals are the only people qualified to give you answers.
6. Your emotional and physical well-being depend on how intelligently you handle yourself in this medical crisis. Beating breast cancer means finding it early, receiving quality treatment, and diligent follow-up.

PART FOUR

The Real Costs— Emotional and Financial

CHAPTER 12

....

Gathering Support

Rebecca: When a woman is confronted with a life-threatening illness, such as breast cancer, her priorities change. What was important yesterday is inconsequential today. There are so many factors involved in treating breast cancer. You begin to feel as if you have to be superwoman to accommodate your normal work load in addition to the burdens of seeking an appropriate diagnosis. You wonder if you are up to coping with the demands made upon you. Can you handle the fear and the emotions of those who love you—your husband, your children, your parents, your friends? The answer is that you can and you do deal with this emotional and physical trauma.

The question is how successfully do you deal with it? The women who adjust successfully to the breast cancer diagnosis and its treatment have respect for their well-being; they are aggressive in seeking the best possible treatment available; and, they rely on those around them who can and do give emotional support.

Women in general have very little concrete information about breast cancer and a wealth of misinformation about the disease. Unless a person or family has been touched by "cancer," most people are frightened by the very word. People behave differently when confronted with a cancer diagnosis. Some women attack the problem with intense discipline—reading, calling, asking questions, searching for answers. Those women need to control the situation. Other women, however, repress their fears and emotions; they deny or minimize the importance of the diagnosis; and some of them fail altogether to confront the issue.

Regardless of your personality type, you should try to remain focused on your breast cancer diagnosis so that you can accomplish your goal of seeking treatment appropriate for you. For instance, if you minimize the impact of your breast cancer, you are not going to be aggressive in searching for the best possible doctors and facilities. On the other hand, if you plan an all-out attack you can subject yourself to unnecessary pressure above and beyond normal objectivity. Obviously, a middle-of-the-road approach is most useful. This will allow you to accumulate the information that will help you make an intelligent decision without creating extreme stress.

Once you are confronted with a diagnosis you will be amazed at the amount of time cancer requires. The research, the scheduling of medical tests, the consultations—they all require significant amounts of preparation time. This can be a catharsis in and of itself. After the diagnosis some women stick to their work and social schedules while others find that impossible to do. While one woman may adopt an attitude of powerlessness, another will overcome her fear with strength and authority. A woman must follow her own instincts to help her cope with the physical and emotional aspects that generally come with the initial discovery that she has breast cancer. It is within all of us to accept the challenge of the demands of the disease made upon us at this time.

I found it amazing at how easily women can adjust to the physical demands of breast cancer; the psychological demands, however, are another matter. We seem to have remarkable resilience and most of us have the ability to overcome such assaults to our psyche. Being involved in the health-care process gives us a sense that we are doing something positive in the management of our life and of our breast cancer.

I am always impressed with the women I have met who are able to cope with the demands of breast cancer while maintaining a good sense of humor. A positive mental state is necessary to keep a sense of balance in our lives. While it is key to maintaining perspective in our personal and professional relationships, it also makes us better patients. Adopting a positive attitude can see us through those pressured and emotional periods that we encounter as we deal with our diagnosis. Cancer is so much more than a physical disease. It tests those emotions related to our well-being, our core, our soul.

To manage the breast cancer diagnosis you have to share it with the appropriate people in your life who are equipped to give you the most support. I felt most fortunate to have had the support of a loving husband, two parents who were there for me, a beautiful sister and brother who were truly helpful, and a teenage son who with his own busy life offered me diversion from medical stress. The most blessed gift we can have in our lives is to have a special person with whom we can share life's tragedies. For some that may be a husband, or family member, or a trusted friend, or a God. If we are truly fortunate we have all of them to lend their support, their strength, and their love. Women seem to recover much more quickly both physically and emotionally when there are concerned and supportive people around them.

In a trusting personal relationship we can share our fears about death, discuss the quality of our lives, and provide us with an outlet so that we can temporarily give in to the grief that we feel. It is important to spend some time thinking about the injustice of what has happened so that you can free yourself from the psychological hold that cancer has upon you. Only then can you move forward toward your goal of conquering the disease.

Breast cancer is a disease that is so tied to our feminine identity that we can lose all perspective on what it actually means to our body as a whole. Because most of us have spent our lives trying to make the best of what nature had given us, the thought of breast cancer terrifies us. We are quickly forced to reevaluate just how much importance is placed on our appearance. Unfortunately, we tend to think in terms of how a partner or mate will view us rather than making an objective personal assessment. Honest communication between partners should positively reinforce the relationship and enable you to clarify your goals.

This is a time when you will appreciate a closeness with

your children and family. While we all want to protect our children from pain and unhappiness, it is important to be forthright with them about your illness. The more they have an understanding of what is happening to you the less frightened they will be. My fourteen-year-old son was away at boarding school for the period I was on chemotherapy. One day the school nurse took me aside to ask me how I was doing. She said she had a student whose mother was going through treatment for breast cancer and he wasn't handling it well. His grades were suffering, he was having peer problems and was troubled. I can only assume that his mother wanted to distance him from her illness. It just doesn't work with older children. They become more frightened from not knowing.

If your child is a teenager, this is a period when they are struggling with their own sexual identity, and the focus on your breasts can be unsettling to them. Once again, your attitude will determine how successfully they deal with your having cancer—they take their direction from you. It is heartening to see how much you mean to them and how they will try to make your ordeal easier. They will surprise you with their ability to cope.

News travels fast when you have a diagnosis of breast cancer. The unsettling nature of all cancers, especially breast cancer, only intensifies the anxiety of the people around you who know what you are going through. We are viewed by some people as unhealthy, plagued, or worse, to be pitied. The general public assumes that we are living with a death sentence. It is difficult to believe that in the 1990s this subject can provoke these feelings. I am amazed that public perception can be so outdated.

Dealing with friends, acquaintances, and business associates can be disturbing too. It is difficult for some people to find the right words without being solicitous. You will receive calls from people you haven't spoken to in years. You will also not hear from people you thought you knew quite well. You will experience the pain of having a friend who is uncomfortable with you or worse, has abandoned you, upon hearing of your illness. They will not only avoid you, they will be gone from your life. Of course your true friends are just that, true friends.

However, some people will be extremely uncomfortable that you have breast cancer. It can be distressing to have people around you who try to force cheerfulness. Others just don't want to acknowledge or talk about your disease, and you aren't sure whether they are afraid for themselves or for you. In time, however, those people usually choose to forget your illness.

Dr. Petrek: Group therapy and support groups can be very helpful to the newly diagnosed woman. Being in contact with women who have the same symptoms or are experiencing the same treatment can be helpful. Self-help groups are available where women can obtain concrete information, share experiences, and gather hope. There are people who want to talk to you about your cancer and are in a position to help you. They may be interested because of a mother, aunt, or friend who has had breast cancer, or perhaps they personally have had a scare. Many therapists have had breast cancer themselves and understand the emotions that surface when one is searching for treatment and cure. Being with women who are coping well with their disease can have a positive influence on you. While participation in support groups usually occurs after breast surgery and during follow-up treatment, a telephone call to a breast cancer support organization can yield valuable information when approaching a surgical decision.

Rebecca: Most communities have some type of information and support network for current patients with breast cancer. To locate organizations in your area you can call your local or state chapter of the American Cancer Society, listed in the Part Five Database, or one of the Comprehensive Cancer Centers in your region. You can also call a hospital in your area and ask what they have available for breast cancer information. You can also call national organizations such as the National Alliance of Breast Cancer Organizations (NABCO) 212-719-0154; SHARE: Self-Help for Women with Breast Cancer at 212-382-2111; Y-ME National Organization for Breast Cancer Information and Support at 800-221-2141; and The YWCA Encore Program at 212-614-2827 for help in locating local sources of information.

For some women the best way of dealing with their cancer is to talk about it. But other women wish to keep the disease to themselves and a few people close to them. It is a personal decision about whom you will share this information with, either family and close friends or a network of individuals. It can sometimes be difficult to express your true feelings, because people want to see you with a positive attitude; they are more comfortable when you are coping well. It is important, however, to have a friend with whom you can be totally honest. Sharing fears and concerns, outrage, and sadness with a close friend is good for both of you.

Dr. Petrek: There has been so much written lately about the body as it relates to the mind and the mind as it relates to the body. It is a terrible responsibility to carry with you the guilt that you might have caused your cancer by personal neglect or a negative mind-set. I personally believe that the development of breast cancer is not influenced by personality type or stress. Other doctors believe that it might be.

What we can do is change our habits from now on to help live long and healthy lives. Of course, there is the mistaken attitude that you can cure your own illness through proper diet, exercise, positive thinking, and mind management techniques. This is a lifelong burden of responsibility. Don't fall into a "guilt gully" and blame yourself for the cancer. You did not cause your breast cancer, and you cannot cure the disease without sound medical assistance.

Rebecca: At the same time, as you are sorting through your emotions regarding your breast cancer, don't neglect your body. Review the cancer lifestyle profiles and the risk patterns that were outlined in chapter 7. If you haven't been living a "healthy lifestyle," now is a good time to start. There is nothing like a cancer diagnosis to make you more aware of responsible living habits. Hopefully, we have eliminated excesses such as tobacco and alcohol, and we are controlling what stresses we do have. We should incorporate into our lives a healthful and varied diet that includes the necessary nutrients and vitamins. Cut down on salt, sugar, and fats. A healthy body can stand up to the anxiety and tension that you are living with now better than a body deficient in basic nutrients.

If you have been exercising prior to your cancer diagnosis, continue to do so. If you do not have a regular exercise regimen, now is a good time to start as you will have two to four weeks between biopsy and surgery. This is enough time to begin a simple walking program that can increase your fitness, tone your tissues, and promote good circulation in your heart and blood vessels. This can take the form of a neighborhood walk, an exercise class at your health club, or jumping to the latest exercise videos.

Exercise will not only help in relieving the stress associated with preparing for your surgery, but it will put your body into better condition at the time of your surgery. I remember the nurse coming into my room just prior to surgery to give me a sedative. As she plunged the needle into my bottom she said, "You are in good shape. You can't imagine the soft buttocks I usually encounter."

Get the required amount of sleep. A refreshed mind and body will serve you better than being nervous and tense from exhaustion. Engage in techniques to encourage relaxation; deep breathing, a distracting project, meditation, a short walk, or simply a soak in the tub can do wonders to reduce tension.

While it is difficult, take time for pleasurable activities. Treat yourself to dinner at your favorite restaurant, go to a movie you have been wanting to see, buy something special for yourself. Take time to do whatever will give you pleasure. Happiness is important to our psychological well-being, and when we are happy we have reduced the level of stress, at least temporarily.

Take this opportunity and use this time to gather spiritual strength. If you are one of the fortunate who is comfortable with God, you will no doubt question the confirming diagnosis. And it takes great strength to overcome the power of doubt. You need not travel this road alone. You may discover that your spiritual life has improved as a result of your cancer and that can give you a certain peace to help you cope with your disease.

Finally, there are almost always positive results to your having breast cancer. For instance, you might have a greater appreciation of family and friends as you see how they have helped you. You now have a healthy respect for your body, and you know you will take better care of it. You have developed a sense that life really is precious and you have taken it for granted for too long. You can identify and eliminate undesirable or insignificant projects from your calendar. You have a renewed faith in yourself and know you will grow personally from having conquered breast cancer.

Your relationship with your spouse or a significant other might also prove more meaningful—the "...in sickness and in health..." line from the marriage vows have been tested. You are much easier on yourself, much less critical and much more accommodating of your imperfections. And you no longer carry around as many unrealistic expectations about your life and your abilities. These can be significant improvements in your life, and the realization is due to your breast cancer diagnosis. In short, paradoxically cancer can help save your life.

CHAPTER CHECKLIST

1. Don't blame yourself. Your body has malfunctioned through no fault of your own.
2. Select a few individuals with whom you can intimately confide. Don't be afraid to rely on others. Sharing your concerns with others is definitely preferable to withdrawal and repression.
3. Determine what are your best coping mechanisms. Who else will you discuss this with? What will you eliminate from your life for the next two months so you can care for yourself?
4. Your ability to cope is directly tied to your attitude about your illness. Eliminate negative or pessimistic thoughts from your mind. This is a time for confidence that you are taking the best possible action in your own defense.
5. Cancer can be a lifesaver. Take stock and bring some positive action into your life.

CHAPTER 13

....

Managing the Finances

Rebecca: The cost of health care in America has been a prominent issue in the news for some time. We all know that we are going to need at some point some type of health-care services, but we don't often think about it until we are forced to because of an illness. There isn't a woman today who hasn't thought about the financial impact if she were diagnosed with breast cancer.

Naturally, the costs of such a disease are important to every woman and her family. You do not want to compromise the quality of your medical treatment because of the cost, but you cannot afford to ignore the financial impact of your treatment either. In this chapter, we will explore some of the issues pertaining to the finances relating to the treatment of breast cancer. You want to solve the business problems associated with breast cancer more efficiently so that you can concentrate on the physical and psychological aspects necessary for successful treatment.

Dr. Petrek: You have already had the benefits of a number of consultations, diagnostic procedures, surgical procedures, and laboratory analyses. All of these services were necessary to diagnose your breast cancer so that you can receive appropriate and complete treatment. But diagnostic tests and procedures can be expensive.

Follow-up services such as professional breast examinations with your surgeon, periodic blood tests, regularly scheduled mammography, and regular gynecological office visits are important for women who have had breast cancer or for those women who are at high risk for developing breast cancer. Even as the demand increases for follow-up services and preventive maintenance, and the technology becomes more sophisticated, we the consumers are responsible for a greater share of those costs.

Rebecca: Because medical costs have been increasing annually, employers have been forced to transfer a portion of these higher costs to their employees. Most of us have felt the financial pressure of paying a larger share of our medical expenses. In addition, our insurers at times do not cover certain costs connected with our medical treatment. Women in treatment for breast cancer could be forced to deal with medical expenses that their insurance plans will not cover. And, for those without insurance the financial impact can be devastating.

Dr. Petrek: The cost of breast cancer treatments can differ by geographic locations. Unfortunately, no regulations govern the establishment of standardized fees, and the difference in the costs of breast treatment can vary greatly in different parts of the country. For instance, the costs of office space, staff and technician salaries, malpractice insurance, and imaging equipment can all have an effect on treatment costs, and they are usually higher in urban areas.

In a metropolitan area, you have a choice of breast specialists and you can easily compare the fees that they charge with the services they provide. Doctors know that they are competing with other specialists for your business and they don't want to lose you as a patient so their fees are usually competitive. If you are in an area where there are few qualified breast specialists, however, you might want to consider going to a larger city or regional medical facility and pay the cost differential.

Rebecca: For many women, questioning a doctor about his fees is uncomfortable, and many don't even bother to ask. It is a question that doctors expect the patients to ask their secretary, and a good specialist will be prepared to respond specifically about the charges. The doctor should also be able to give you an estimate of the costs of any additional treatment or therapy. If you can't deal with fee discussions, have a family member or friend with you during the consultation to bring up the matter. Remember, medicine is big business with the same economic incentives as any other type of business.

The medical profession is aware of the economic limitations on some families. In some cases the fees may be adjusted upward or downward depending on your ability to pay. Doctors, for instance, can and often do lower their fees so that they are in line with what your insurance will pay. Insurers very often will be able to help you in negotiating more favorable rates for physicians and hospital services. Moreover, the hospital that you select may have a Financial Representative or Patient Account Services who can help you find other resources if you qualify for financial need. In other words, negotiation is possible, and there may be other financial options available, so don't be uncomfortable asking about financial matters.

The billing and payment of medical services in a clinic or a hospital is generally taken care of in one of several ways. The hospital can bill your insurer directly, you may pay on a fee-for-service basis and have your insurer reimburse you for the expense, or you may pay a portion of the bill and have the remainder billed to your insurer. Each time a medical service is performed, either a physician visit, a laboratory test, or a diagnostic or surgical procedure, a fee is charged. You could be responsible for payment of any fees or charges, and you should be prepared to do so each time you use a medical service. Payment is usually expected before you leave the medical facility.

Unfortunately, no package deal or all-inclusive fee is available for breast cancer treatment. Services are expensed as they are provided, and mistakes in the billing can occur. Usually every doctor's office has a specific employee responsible for the billing and to deal with the variety of insurers and health-care plans. In planning her treatment, a patient can meet with an office manager or a financial counselor at the hospital or clinic to discuss the costs associated with her individual breast cancer.

Many large corporate employers have on staff, or are retaining, cost-management specialists to review insurance claims and monitor requests for major tests, procedures, and services. Your company may also have an employee-benefits manager who can help you in determining what are "reasonable and customary" fees. In an effort to control expenses, they look for questionable diagnostic tests and unnecessary or inappropriate procedures and medical services. They can be of great help to you in trying to sift through what is appropriate and cost-effective in breast cancer treatment.

As an informed medical consumer, it makes good sense to know exactly what you are paying for and who will be responsible for the payment. Each time you schedule an appointment for a consultation, test, scan, or any medical service, you should ask the cost, the method of payment, and when you need to pay for the service. Each time you receive a medical service, make sure you have the required method of payment ready; cash, credit card, checks, and insurance reimbursement forms.

The complicated and extensive paperwork on the costs and insurances involved in breast cancer treatment require diligent record keeping. You will want to have a master file with current insurance documents, personnel and employer correspondence updates, and any pertinent financial information available for immediate access and reference. Organize your bills and payments in a file to cross-check what services have been performed, what you have paid, and what is in process for insurance or employer reimbursement.

FINANCIAL CHECKLIST

1. What is the fee for this test, consultation? What does it include? Do they bill separately for each procedure? Will there be additional expenses? What will they be? Make sure you have other test results available to avoid duplication of the same test. Is the fee in line with what your insurance will cover? Will they accept the amount your insurance covers as full payment? Has an insurance company ever recommended nonpayment of their fee?

2. Call the hospital you are considering and ask for a fee schedule. What does it include? What are their billing practices? Do they itemize their bills? Do they charge

separately for services? Will they bill your insurance directly?

3. Call the insurance company to determine what tests, procedures, medical fees, and hospitalizations are covered under your policy. Get a price range from them on what is reasonable and customary. Will they require approval prior to your surgery?

4. Ask your insurer if they retain a cost-management consultant who can help you identify unnecessary or costly procedures. From this cost range you can estimate what your financial responsibility will be. They can also be helpful in leading you to more cost-efficient doctors and hospitals.

5. Most insurers or HMO's have human resources personnel to offer you administrative support to help in evaluating the costs of your breast cancer. They may be helpful in negotiating discounted fees.

6. If you have an open-ended insurer plan, ask what the base fee is that you need to pay. What is the deductible? What is the copayment? What about the remainder? Is there a cap or maximum on what they will cover? Is the limit for each medical service or the total?

The Cancer Spreadsheet

The cancer spreadsheet is an analysis of the costs commonly associated with treatment for breast cancer. The costs have been separated into categories expensed as they might have occurred in the Strategic Lifeline in chapter 2. The categories are coded according to the function of medical service performed: consultations, diagnostic tests, pathology and laboratory services, interpretation of the diagnostic and laboratory tests, hospital expenses, physician services, medications, and follow-up.

As you scan the cost estimates, at first glance you will be shocked at the amount of money that can be spent on treatments for breast cancer. Keep two things in mind when evaluating these costs. First, because there are a variety of treatment options for breast cancer, not all of the services will be recommended for you. And second, the Cost Ranges are just that, approximate ranges. Costs can vary according the location, type of facility, and the individual physician. The cost estimates were compiled from several sources: a small city hospital, a regional medical center between two rural states, and a large city cancer center. For instance, fees could be considerably higher in an urban situation than in a rural or suburban region. Consider both factors when using the cost analysis as a basis for your own breast cancer expenses.

ANALYSIS OF THE COSTS OF BREAST CANCER*

C-Consultation   M-Medication
D-Diagnostic Test   MD-Doctor Services
F-Follow-up   P-Pathology and Laboratory
H-Hospital   S-Surgical
I-Interpretation

*All fees quoted are one-time fee-for-service charges

PREDIAGNOSIS	CODE	COST RANGE
Gynecologist	C	$75–175
Mammogram (bilateral)	D	75–200
Ultrasound (unilateral)	D	75–250
Breast Surgeon	C	100–350
Needle Biopsy	D	150–400
Specimen Analysis	P	75–120

SURGICAL BIOPSY		
Hospital	H	$1,000–1,500
Surgeon	MD	1,500–2,500
Anesthesiologist	MD	400–750
Presurgical Preparation	H	200–300
Chest X ray	D	60–150
Read X ray results	I	30–50
EKG	D	45–200
Read EKG results	I	30–50
Blood Workup	P	75–150
Tissue Specimen Analysis	P	200–500
Second Opinion Review	P	75–350

ADDITIONAL TESTS		
CAT Scan	D	$500–900
Analyze Results	I	150–300
Bone Scan	D	250–500
Analyze Results	I	100–150
Liver Scan	D	200–300
Analyze Results	I	100–150
MRI	D	600–1,500
Analyze Results	I	150–300

SECOND OPINIONS		
Surgeon #2	C	$100–350
Surgeon #3	C	100–350
Oncologist	C	150–400
Radiologist	C	150–450
Plastic Surgeon	C	150–250
Cancer Specialist	C	150–500

SURGERIES (INCLUDING SURGEONS' FEES)	CODE	COST RANGE
Excisional Biopsy	S	$1,200–1,800
Excisional Biopsy with Preop. needle localization	S	1,750–2,250
Stereo Core Biopsy	S	1,500–2,000
Lumpectomy	S	1,600–2,000
Lumpectomy with Preop. needle localization	S	2,400–3,000
Lumpectomy with Axillary Dissection	S	4,000–6,000
Simple Mastectomy	S	2,600–3,200
Modified Radical Mastectomy with Axillary Dissection	S	4,500–8,000
Modified Radical Mastectomy with Axillary Dissection and immediate breast reconstruction	S	5,500–9,000
Bilateral Mastectomy with two Axillary Dissections	S	6,500–10,000
Breast Reconstruction		
Expander Implant	S	5,000–7,000
Implant	S	4,000–6,000
Tissue Transfer	S	7,000–15,000
Nipple	S	2,000–5,000
RADIATION THERAPY		
Treatment Planning	H	$300–800
Mold & Simulation	H	250–350
Initial Films	D	80–250
Radiation Treatment cost per session		
35 sessions	H	200–450
Full treatment	H	7,000–15,750
Physician Checkup		
Full treatment	MD	350–700
Weekly	MD	50–100
Miscellaneous Expenses*	H	275–400

*Additional X rays, blood counts, and physician support

CHEMOTHERAPY-Six Months

	CODE	COST RANGE	TIME	
Physician Checkup	MD	$900–1,800	Bimonthly	75–150
Physician Supervision	MD	900–1,200	Bimonthly	75–100
Treatment	H	1,200–3,600	Bimonthly	100–300
Weekly Blood Counts	P	960–1,440	Weekly	40–60
Blood Analysis	P	1,920–2,800	Weekly	80–120
Pharmaceuticals	M	450–600	Monthly	75–100
Miscellaneous Expenses**	H	200–250		

**Additional blood workups

FOLLOW-UP

	CODE	COST RANGE	TIME	
Physical Examination	MD		***	
Surgeon		$75–225	3-2-1	
Radiologist		75–175	3-2-1	
Oncologist		75–250	4-3-2-1	
Mammogram bilateral)	D	75–200	2-2-1	
Blood Workup	P	40–60	4-3-2-1	
Laboratory analysis	P	80–120	4-3-2-1	
Chest X ray	D	60–150	1	
Read X ray	I	30–50	1	
Physical Therapy	F	75–300		
Lymphedema	F	130–250		
Hormone Therapy-Tamoxifen	F	100–200	Monthly	
		1,200–2,000	Annual	
Breast Reconstruction				
Plastic Surgeon Con- sultation	MD	200–350		

***4, 3, 2, 1 means appointments annually for years 1–5 +

HOSPITAL CHARGES	CODE	COST RANGE
Preadmission Procedures	H	$200–300
EKG	D	50–200
EKG Analysis	I	30–50
Chest X ray	D	60–150
X ray Analysis	I	30–50
Hospital Room	H	1,800–3,000
3 days @ $600–1,000/day		
Operating Room	H	1,500–2,500
Recovery Room	H	400–750
Anesthesiologist	MD	1,000–1,500
Miscellaneous Expenses*	H	400–700

PATHOLOGY AND LABORATORY SERVICES

Tissue Specimen	P	$400–700
Tissue Analysis	I	350–600
Frozen-Section Specimen	P	200–300
Frozen-Section Analysis	I	100–175
DNA Flow Test	P	175–400

POSTSURGICAL EXPENSES

Pharmaceuticals	M	$75–125
Postsurgical Checkup	MD	60–95

*Miscellaneous expenses can include: IV therapy, medical and surgical supplies, pharmaceuticals, blood work, physical therapy, and telephone

CHAPTER 14

....

Managing the Insurance

Rebecca: So many types of insurance are available today, and when we are faced with a breast cancer diagnosis we come to realize just how important their role is in the quality of our treatment. It is important for you to know if your insurer will provide adequate and effective coverage for your breast cancer treatment. Whether your insurer is Medicare, Medicaid, a commercial insurance carrier, a Blue Cross/Blue Shield plan, a group health insurer, a health maintenance organization (HMO), a preferred-provider organization (PPO), individual practice association (IPA), a point-of-service system (POS), or you are self-insured, you have a right to expect at least partial payment for the costs incurred in a breast cancer diagnosis and treatment plan.

Dr. Petrek: Regardless of what type of national health care plan is devised, it won't be implemented for several years and you are in the position of having to work with the insurer that presently provides your coverage. The first step is to find the insurance policy or medical plan booklet, read it, and make an effort to understand exactly what benefits you are eligible to receive. Most plans have a pamphlet that describes the plan and its requirements for effective use. This will not be an easy task but one that is necessary and should be done before you schedule the diagnostic tests for breast cancer.

Certain medical plans may be structured differently but they all contain:

1. A summary of health care facts and benefits that

outline what your plan covers and what you must do to receive those benefits.

2. An enrollment application or contract that will specify the date your actual coverage begins and can tell you if there is a waiting period before you are qualified to receive benefits.

3. A contribution schedule with your monthly, quarterly, semiannual, or annual fee rates.

4. A description of medical services along with deductible expenses and copayment responsibilities to determine what you must pay before the plan becomes effective. This should also define the maximum dollar amount on specific benefits that the policy will pay over your lifetime.

5. A list of limitations and exclusions. Read this carefully. Does it mention preexisting conditions or specifically cancer?

6. A list of your rights and responsibilities as a member of the health plan or the insured.

7. A description of the process and procedures in filing claims.

8. Correspondence on updates and changes in coverage since you have enrolled in the plan.

As you review the insurance policy or health plan, you should begin to formulate a list of questions to ask when you call your insurer. The chapter checklist will suggest questions that you might want to ask. Each plan will have its specific limitations and restrictions on surgeries, treatments, and drugs, and you want to determine that your treatment will be covered.

Once your physician has determined that you in fact do have a suspicious lump you should call your insurer or health plan. For many women this may be the first contact that they have had with their insurer and it may take a few telephone calls to connect with a person who can help them. In some plans the title of the person is the Managed Care professional, but for other insurers it may be the Benefits Provider, Member Service Representative, or a Claims Agent. Most plans, however, require that you call first when you are considering a hospital admission with accompanying surgical procedure in order to receive the full plan benefits. Call promptly. A delay might possibly jeopardize certain reimbursements.

There are a number of reasons why the insurer is one of the first calls that you make in connection with a possible breast cancer diagnosis. First, you want to determine what their recommended procedure is for investigating a possible breast cancer. For instance, if mammography is recommended will they make payment even though you may have had a prior mammogram only a few months ago? Do they reimburse for ultrasound? What about the costs of a biopsy? Should it be performed in a clinic or must you be hospitalized?

Second, you want to have an estimate of costs connected with the diagnosis. You want to know how much each diagnostic test and procedure should cost and what your deductible or copayment will be. You want to know if there is a limit beyond which you are responsible for any additional costs.

Third, you may need their approval for any second opinion consultations you might need. Ask if there are specific breast surgeons that the insurer recommends. Are they board-certified? What are their typical breast surgical fees?

And fourth, you will want to know the procedure for processing claims. You will also want to know if they expect you to notify them as expenses are incurred or what, if any, additional follow-up contact is necessary.

The amount of paperwork generated when seeking a diagnosis of breast cancer can be overwhelming. To make your insurance reimbursement and bill-paying more efficient you may want to organize your receipts, bills, and claim forms in separate file folders. You will need a folder for those claims that are not yet submitted to your insurer, and a folder for the receipts for those expenses that are to be billed directly to your insurer, and a folder for those claims that are in process. Hospital business offices and doctors occasionally make mistakes, and duplicate billing is quite common in the medical community. You will save a great deal of time if you can locate bills and receipts quickly.

Don't forget to keep a record of any miscellaneous expenses incurred as a result of your breast cancer diagnosis, such as automobile expenses, meals, taxi, copying, and unreimbursed small medical bills. An itemized account of your expenses may be needed for tax purposes, and you will be relieved not to have to reconstruct a list of expenses at tax time.

If you have no insurance and in the past have paid for medical services as they were provided you still should expect to receive good-quality treatment for your breast cancer. For inpatient hospitalizations you will probably be expected to pay a deposit to secure your room, and when you are released the hospital may require complete payment of your final bill. If you cannot meet your financial obligation to the hospital and can prove financial need, you can request to speak to an Account Representative to assist you in seeking other methods of payment. They may be able to provide you with emergency alternatives to help with the costs. Most hospitals take cash, checks, money orders, and most of the usual credit cards.

For those women who are uninsured because of economic circumstances there are several organizations that can help you obtain a good breast cancer diagnosis and the necessary treatment. You can ask your local chapter of the American Cancer Society to recommend low-cost mammography facilities, to suggest a breast surgeon who perhaps has a limited practice of patients in need, and recommend hospitals that are more lenient in offering treatment to the uninsured. Call your state's insurance commissioner, and ask if there are laws that can give uninsured residents access to health insurance. Also state and government health agencies can and will subsidize health insurance coverage for needy patients. In addition, certain private health-care organizations have access to financial aid that can help you in finding good quality treatment. Refer to the Database in Part Five for information in your region.

As more and more women survive early breast cancer treatment there are a number of insurance issues that they can encounter as they resume normal lives. Some may relate to your situation and some may not. However, you should be aware that you could possibly encounter social censure, employment discrimination, and health insurance injustices.

Some women may discover that their choice of doctors, hospitals, and treatments could be decreassed by their health plan because they have a diagnosis of breast cancer. Companies can and do reduce reimbursment if an employee chooses a doctor outside their list of recommended specialists. Some health-care plans have a limited list of specialty medical professionals, and a woman may be forced to look beyond the list of doctors her insurer suggests in seeking appropriate treatment.

It is unfortunate that while you are dealing with a diagnosis of cancer you may also discover the not-so-pleasant details of your health plan. It is important to understand the limitations and restrictions prior to your surgery so that there will be no surprises during or after treatment. A preexisting condition, such as breast cancer, can mean that some women could be excluded from certain insurance coverages at a later date, even if her cancer is considered to be cured.

You could be rejected by some insurers if you change jobs or retire without maintaining your insurance coverage. There can be significant differences in coverage when you do change jobs. Some group policies very often are not transferable to another employer, so you may be forced to stay in a difficult employment situation until you are able to find another insurer.

Federal and state laws now forbid dismissal of an employee based on the employee's medical history. The Americans with Disabilities Act, effective in July of 1992, prohibits employment discrimination by employers against people with disabilities. The word disability is defined broadly to include people who are perceived as having a disability or some past disability, including breast cancer.

A federal law known as COBRA (Consolidated Omnibus Budget Reconciliation Act) now requires that your employer offer you the opportunity to continue your existing group coverage for 18 months after you have left their employ. As long as you pay your monthly premiums you will need to pay only a nominal fee in addition to what the company paid for your coverage.

Seeking insurance can be time-consuming but finding alternative coverage will give the woman facing a possible breast cancer diagnosis, added financial and medical security. Breast cancer diagnosis and treatment should not prevent you from fulfilling your employment obligations or obtaining adequate insurance.

The final problem issue in insurance has to do with your medical history record. The word cancer in a medical or professional file, even if the cancer has been in remission or considered cured, could mean that you could pay higher insurance premiums, or worse, be denied future coverage. Some insurers will not reimburse claims because the breast cancer had already been diagnosed prior to the existing coverage.

Other health plans may not cover a woman with a previous diagnosis of breast cancer at all. At a recent lecture on health insurance issues at one of this country's leading cancer centers, several patients told horror stories about inadequate or nonexistent payments for regularly prescribed cancer treatments.

Where does this medical information come from, and who needs access to it anyway? Think about the number of times you fill out forms that ask for specific information about you—your social security number, your employer, your bank, your credit cards, the state of your health, your insurer, etc. We are frequently asked to sign forms to release personal information without really knowing who is requesting this information and what they are doing with it. As a result, corporations, businesses, banks, insurance companies, HMO's, state and federal government organizations, the courts, public service agencies, educational institutions, and anyone with the right computer connections can have access to our medical records.

You need to question the validity of those who request personal information about you and your breast cancer. You will want to know how protective the hospital is of your health records. Do they respect your privacy? You can obtain a copy of your medical profile from the Medical Information Bureau (617-426-3660) to verify the accuracy of their information. Errors do occur, and it could jeopardize future insurance coverage. If the MIB has a file on you it should be accurate, and it could help if you are involved in an employment or discrimination problem.

INSURANCE CHECKLIST

1. Contact your insurer. You want to know what their procedure is for investigating a possible breast cancer. What is covered in a breast cancer diagnosis?
2. What are the cost ranges for tests and procedures? What is your deductible or copayment percentage? Is there a cap or maximum limit to what the plan pays? Are you fully responsible thereafter?
3. What is their procedure for processing claims? What should you do to follow-up with them?
4. Can they recommend one or two breast surgeons in your area? Are they board-certified? What are their typical surgical fees?
5. Call your state insurance commissioner to find out if there is legislation that will protect you if you do not have insurance. Ask for the names of companies that will provide insurance for high-risk or uninsurable people.
6. Does your insurance company have a flexible benefits plan? Is the policy guaranteed to be renewable? Can they cancel it at will? Can you continue coverage if you leave? Is there an alternative individual plan available for you to convert to should you be terminated either through divorce or death of a spouse?
7. Obtain a copy of your health insurance profile from the Medical Information Bureau (617-426-3660). Also, secure a copy of your hospital records. Both documents will give you ammunition if you are confronted by a discriminatory employer or insurer.
8. Keep a complete inventory of your bills, receipts, and claims. The documentation will be helpful in the event of an error.

CHAPTER 15

Conclusion: Making the Decision

We make decisions all our lives, in a variety of different circumstances, under many different conditions. As mature, adult women, making decisions is a function of the busy lives that we lead. Some of the decisions that we must make are relatively unimportant. Once the decision has been made and then acted upon it is forgotten. Other decisions, however, have a significant and lasting impact on our lives. Regardless of the type of decision we must make, some of us enjoy the challenge of the decision-making process, while many others will do anything to avoid making a decision.

Taking responsibility for our own health care involves making many decisions. Dealing with a breast cancer diagnosis and then ultimately deciding on your medical treatment can be frightening but also empowering. Frightening because you will have consulted with many medical experts and probably spent hundreds if not thousands of dollars in the course of determining your breast cancer diagnosis. But, for all the time and expense, the experts won't tell you what you should do, they will only make recommendations. And, if you have had second and third opinion consultations, you may have two or three different treatment recommendations. What do you do?

Clearly you need to analyze and possibly improve on your decision-making skills. How do you do this so that you can confidently make the treatment decision that is appropriate for you?

DECISION CHECKLIST

1. Review the successful and positive decisions you have made in the past. Ask yourself what learning processes enabled you to make those important decisions. Had you studied the problem? Did you seek out the advice of trusted friends, colleagues or advisors? Acknowledging that you have made good decisions previously will reinforce the fact that you have the ability to continue to do so.

2. Think of your breast cancer in the long term. This may sound obvious but so many women become trapped by not thinking that there is life after breast cancer. The decisions that you make now should be based on the best information and treatment technology presently available. Your future peace of mind will depend on this.

3. Remain focused on the results of your breast cancer diagnosis. This will be easy because you won't be thinking of much else. However, you don't want to feel pressured or influenced by the fears of other people so that you postpone taking the necessary positive action that is appropriate for you.

4. Recognize when you have accumulated enough information to make a conscientious decision. You don't need to become an expert in breast cancer, but you do want sufficient medical information to feel comfortable making choices for your type of cancer.

5. Keep an open mind about the treatment options recommended to you. Don't give in to the preconceptions you might have had about breast cancer prior to your diagnosis. You are much better informed now and should feel confident about your choices.

6. Trust your own good instincts. Only you can evaluate your emotions, your personal relationships, your business, your lifestyle, and your family situation. These nonmedical situations have a bearing on your decision-making process. Make the decision based on what is best for you.

7. Set aside some quality time just for yourself to relax and contemplate what is happening to you. Important decisions cannot be made when your mind is filled with confusing

and conflicting information. If you can relieve the nervous tension that seems to overwhelm you during the breast cancer diagnosis, you will probably discover that the right decision for you will become clear.

8. Finally, don't second-guess yourself. Once you have made the decision as to what treatment is going to be appropriate for you, take the positive action necessary to implement that decision. Have the confidence to proceed with your treatment and follow-up according to what you and your doctor have jointly agreed upon.

PART FIVE

....

A Database of Sources and Resources

The Database consists of five major sections. The first and largest section is a state-by-state listing organized in eight regions nationwide. Included in each state list is the address of that state's division of the American Cancer Society, the name and location of a National Cancer Institute (NCI) Comprehensive Cancer Center, and the name and address of state agencies that deal with health-related issues such as administering health care programs, Medicare and Medicaid services, medical licensing, insurance regulations, services for the aging, and women's commissions or other human resources.

Not all state agencies are uniformly titled. For instance, the Department of Occupational and Professional Licensing may be listed under the Office of Consumer Affairs in one state but be listed under the Department of Health and Welfare in another state. For each state you will find a telephone number to call for verification of medical professionals, sites, and services.

The American Cancer Society has a wealth of written information on breast cancer as well as other types of cancers, and their Public Information Department is a logical conduit to locating local and regional medical professionals, hospitals, clinics, support groups, and other public services. There may not be a National Cancer Institute (NCI) Comprehensive Cancer Center in your state, but there will be one in your region or in an adjoining state. Cross-reference the states to locate the larger clinics and medical centers.

Section Two is a listing of national organizations and associations equipped to provide you with information of all types relating to breast cancer. Some have 800 numbers or hotlines so that you can receive information quickly.

Section Three lists national organizations, associations, and government agencies that can help with the business aspects of breast cancer. These include information on insurances, financial assistance, verification of facilities, retrieval of medical records, and public advocacy groups to help with problem issues.

Section Four contains a list of medical boards and associations that in some instances can provide you with literature and reports on breast cancer. Some medical associations will provide you with a list of board-certified physician specialists in your area. You can also call to verify a physician's board certification.

Section Five is a listing of reference books that may be found in your local library. Recognizing that all local libraries are not created equal, you may find a more extensive reference collection in your county library or your state medical library. Most, however, will have some type of information on breast cancer that will be useful to you.

While we have not listed specific titles of books on breast cancer, the bibliography contains many good sources available. A larger chain bookstore, a specialized medical bookstore, or a university bookstore will have the greatest selection to choose from. Many excellent health newsletters are published by leading medical institutions in which you will find articles dealing with breast cancer. For more technical information, the leading medical journals published by the larger medical societies also have articles of interest on breast cancer.

Many good local organizations provide both information and support to women facing a breast cancer diagnosis. Your state division of the American Cancer Society can provide you with the names and locations of groups in your area. The National Alliance of Breast Cancer Organizations (NABCO) prints an extensive listing of local support organizations nationwide. It is a complete resource list, and I urge you to call NABCO (212-719-0154) to receive a copy.

SECTION ONE

. . . .

A State-by-State Listing

A state-by-state list organized in eight regions nationwide that includes the state division of the American Cancer Society, a NCI Comprehensive Cancer Center either by state or region, and the names and addresses of state agencies that deal with health-related issues.

Region One   Northeast   CT, ME, MA, NH, RI, VT

Region Two   Mid-Atlantic   DE, DC, MD, NJ, NY, PA

Region Three   Southeast   FL, GA, NC, SC, VA, WV

Region Four   Midwest North   IL, IN, IO, MI, MN, OH, WI

Region Five   Midwest South   AL, AR, KY, LA, MS, MO, TN

Region Six   Central North   MT, NE, ND, SD, WY

Region Seven   Central South   AZ, CO, KS, NM, OK, TX, UT

Region Eight   Pacific   AK, CA, HI, NV, OR, WA

Region One / NORTHEAST

....

CONNECTICUT
MAINE
MASSACHUSETTS
NEW HAMPSHIRE
RHODE ISLAND
VERMONT

CONNECTICUT

American Cancer Society
Connecticut Division, Inc.
Barnes Park South
14 Village Lane
Wallingford, CT 06492
203-265-7161

NCI Cancer Center
Yale University
Comprehensive Cancer Center
333 Cedar St., P.O. 3333
New Haven, CT 06510
203-785-6338

State Agency
Department of Aging
Commissioner
175 Main St.
Hartford, CT 06106
203-566-3238

State Agency
Department of Health Services
Commissioner
150 Washington St.
Hartford, Ct 06106
203-566-2038

State Agency
Department of Human
  Resources
Commissioner
1049 Asylum St.
Hartford, CT 06105
203-566-3318

State Agency
Department of Insurance
Commissioner
State Office Building
Hartford, CT 06106
203-297-3802

State Agency
Department of Income
  Maintenance
Medical Care Administrator
110 Bartholomew Ave.
Hartford, Ct 06106
203-566-2934

State Agency
Licensing and Administrative
  Division
Department of Consumer
  Protection
165 Capital Ave.

Hartford, CT 06106
203-566-7177
Medical Quality Assurance
203-566-1482

State Agency
Commission on the Status of
  Women
Commissioner
90 Washington St.
Hartford, CT 06106
203-566-5702

MAINE

American Cancer Society
Maine Division
52 Federal St.
Brunswick, ME 04011
207-729-3339

State Agency
Bureau of Maine's Elderly
Department of Human Services
State House Station #11
Augusta, ME 04333
207-289-2561

State Agency
Department of Human Services
Bureau of Health
State House Station #11
Augusta, ME 04333
207-289-2736

State Agency
Bureau of Insurance
Professional Regulations
  Department
State House Station #34
Augusta, ME 04333
207-289-3101

State Agency
Bureau of Income Maintenance
Department of Human Services
State House Station #11
Augusta, ME 04333
207-289-2415

State Agency
Central Licensing Division
Professional and Financial
  Regulations
State House Station #35
Augusta, ME 04333
207-289-3761

State Agency
Commission for Women
Executive Department
State House Station #93
Augusta, ME 04333
207-289-3417

MASSACHUSETTS

American Cancer Society
Massachusetts Division, Inc.
247 Commonwealth Ave.
Boston, MA 02116
617-267-2650

NCI Cancer Center
Dana Farber Cancer Institute
44 Binney St.
Boston, MA 02115
617-732-3214

State Agency
Executive Office of Elder
  Affairs
Secretary
38 Chauncy St.
Boston, MA 02111
617-727-7750

State Agency
Department of Public Health
Executive Office of Human
  Services
150 Tremont St.
Boston, MA 02111
617-727-2700

State Agency
Executive Office of Human
  Services
Secretary
1 Ashburton Place
Boston, MA 02108
617-727-7600

State Agency
Division of Insurance
Executive Office of Consumer
  Affairs
100 Cambridge St.
Boston, MA 02202
617-727-3357

State Agency
Commissioner Medical
  Payments
Department of Public Walfare
180 Tremont St.
Boston, MA 02111
617-574-0100

State Agency
Division of Registration
Executive Office of Consumer
  Affairs
100 Cambridge St.
Boston, MA 02202
617-727-3074
Registration in Medicine
  617-727-3086

State Agency
Women's Issues
Adviser to Governor
State House, Room 109
Boston, MA 02133
617-727-7853

NEW HAMPSHIRE

American Cancer Society
New Hampshire Division, Inc.
Unit 501
360 Route 101
Bedford, NH 03110
603-472-8899

NCI Cancer Center
Norris Cotton Cancer Center
Dartmouth-Hitchcock Medical
  Center
1 Medical Center Drive
Lebanon, NH 03756
603-650-5000

State Agency
Division of Elderly and Adult
  Services
Department of Health and
  Human Services
Hazen Drive
Concord, NH 03301
603-271-2751

State Agency
Division of Public Health
  Services
Department of Health and
  Welfare
Hazen Drive
Concord, NH 03301
603-271-4505
Medical Board 603-271-4501

State Agency
Division of Human Resources
Office of the Governor
11 Depot St.
Concord, NH 03301
603-271-2611

State Agency
Insurance Department
Commissioner
169 Manchester St.
Concord, NH 03301
603-271-2261

State Agency
Division of Welfare
Department of Health and
  Welfare
Hazen Drive
Concord, NH 03301
603-271-4321

State Agency
Occupational and Professional
  Licensing
Secretary of State
204 State House
Concord, NH 03301
603-271-3242

State Agency
Commission on the Status of
  Women
Chairperson
16 State House Annex
Concord, NH 03301
603-271-2660

RHODE ISLAND

American Cancer Society
Rhode Island Division, Inc.
400 Main St.
Pawtucket, RI 02860
401-722-8480

NCI Cancer Center
Roger Williams Cancer Center
825 Chalkstone Ave.
Providence, RI 02908
401-456-2071

State Agency
Department of Elderly Affairs
Director
79 Washington St.
Providence, RI 02903
401-277-2894

State Agency
Deparmtent of Health
Director
75 Davis St.
Providence, RI 02908
401-277-2231

State Agency
Department of Human Services
Director
600 New London Ave.
Cranston, RI 02920
401-464-2121

State Agency
Department of Business
  Regulation
Director
100 North Main St.
Providence, RI 02903
401-277-2246

State Agency
Medical Services
Dept. of Social and
  Rehabilitation Services
600 New London Ave.
Cranston, RI 02920
401-464-3575

State Agency
Department of Health
Professional Regulation
75 Davis St.
Providence, RI 02908
401-277-2827
Medical Licensing 401-277-2827

State Agency
Department of Labor
Advisory Commission on
  Women
220 Elmwood Ave.
Providence, RI 02907
401-277-2744

VERMONT

American Cancer Society
Vermont Division, Inc.
Drawer C
13 Loomis St.
Montpelier, VT 05602
802-223-2348

NCI Cancer Center
Vermont Cancer Center
University of Vermont
1 South Prospect St.
Burlington, VT 05401
802-656-4580

State Agency
Office on Aging
Agency of Human Services
Waterbury Office Complex
Waterbury, VT 05676
802-241-2400

State Agency
Department of Health
Commissioner
60 Main St.
Burlington, VT 05401
802-863-7280

State Agency
Agency of Human Services
Secretary
103 South Main St.
Waterbury, VT 05676
802-241-2220

State Agency
Department of Insurance and
  Banking
Commissioner
120 State St.
Montpelier, VT 05602
802-828-3301

State Agency
Medical Services Division
Department of Social Welfare
Waterbury Office Complex
Waterbury, VT 05676
802-241-2880

State Agency
Licensing Division
Secretary of State's Office
Redstone
Montpelier, VT 05602
802-828-2363
Medical Practice 802-828-2673
  or 800-642-5155

State Agency
Governor's Commission on the
  Status of Women
Executive Director
126 State St.
Montpelier, VT 05602
802-828-2851

Region Two / MID-ATLANTIC

DELAWARE
DISTRICT OF COLUMBIA
MARYLAND
NEW JERSEY
NEW YORK
PENNSYLVANIA

DELAWARE

American Cancer Society
Delaware Division, Inc.
92 Reads Way, Suite 205
New Castle, DE 19720
302-324-4227

State Agency
Division of Aging
Health and Social Services
  Department
1901 North duPont Highway
New Castle, DE 19720
302-421-6791

State Agency
Division of Public Health
Health and Social Services
  Department
P.O. Box 637, J. Cooper
  Building
Dover, DE 19903
302-736-4701

State Agency
Department of Insurance
The Green
Dover, DE 19901
302-736-4251

State Agency
Division of Economic Services
Health and Social Services
  Department
P.O. Box 906
New Castle, DE 19720
302-421-6139

State Agency
Business and Occupational
  Regulation Division
Administrative Services
  Department
P.O. Box 1401
Dover, DE 19903
302-736-4522

State Agency
Delaware Commission for
  Women
Carvel State Office Building
820 North French Street
Wilmington, DE 19801
302-571-2660

DISTRICT OF COLUMBIA

American Cancer Society
District of Columbia Division,
  Inc.
Suite 315
1825 Connecticut Avenue NW
Washington, DC 20009
202-483-2600

NCI Cancer Center
Lombardi Cancer Research
  Center
Georgetown University Medical
  Center
3800 Reservoir Road NW
Washington, DC 20007
202-687-2192

State Agency
Department of Occupational
  and Professional Licensing
Department of Health and
  Human Services
200 Independence Ave. SW
Washington, DC 20201
202-619-0257
Department of Consumer and
  Regulatory Affairs
202-727-7170

State Agency
Commission for Women
Executive Director
2000 14th St. NW
Washington, DC 20009
202-939-8083

MARYLAND

American Cancer Society
Maryland Division, Inc.
8219 Town Center Drive
Baltimore, MD 21236
410-931-6868

NCI Cancer Center
The Johns Hopkins Oncology
  Center
600 North Wolfe St.
Baltimore, MD 21205
410-955-8638

State Agency
Office on Aging
Room 1004
301 West Preston St.
Baltimore, MD 21201
410-225-1102

State Agency
Department of Health and
  Mental Hygiene
Fifth Floor
201 West Preston St.
Annapolis, MD 21201
410-225-6500

State Agency
Department of Human
  Resources
Secretary
1100 North Eutaw St.
Baltimore, MD 21201
410-333-0001

State Agency
Division of Insurance
Licensing and Regulation
  Department
501 St. Paul St.
Baltimore, MD 21202
410-333-2520

State Agency
Medical Care Programs
Health and Mental Hygiene
  Department
201 West Preston St., Fifth Fl.
Baltimore, MD 21201
410-225-6536

State Agency
Department of Licensing and
  Regulation
Secretary
501 St. Paul Pl.
Baltimore, MD 21202
410-333-6200
Physician Quality Assurance
  301-764-4777

State Agency
Maryland Commission for
  Women
Chairwoman
311 West Saratoga St.
Baltimore, MD 21201
410-767-7137

NEW JERSEY

American Cancer Society
New Jersey Division, Inc.
2600 US Highway 1
North Brunswick, NJ 08902
908-297-8000

State Agency
Division on Aging
Department of Community
  Affairs
363 West State St., CN807
Trenton, NJ 08625
609-292-4833

State Agency
Department of Health
Commissioner
John Fitch Plaza
Trenton, NJ 08625
609-292-7834

State Agency
Department of Human Services
1 Capitol Place
222 South Warren St.
Trenton, NJ 08625
609-292-3717

State Agency
Department of Insurance
Commissioner
20 West State St., 12th Fl.
Trenton, NJ 08625
609-292-5360

State Agency
Division of Medical Assistance
  and Health Services
Department of Human
  Services, CN712
Trenton, NJ 08625
609-588-2600
Medical Examiners
  609-292-4843

State Agency
Division of Consumer Affairs
Department of Law and Public
  Safety
1100 Raymond Blvd., Rm. 504
Newark, NJ 07102
201-648-4010

State Agency
Division on Woman
Department of Community
  Affairs, CN 800
Trenton, NJ 08625
609-292-8840

NEW YORK

American Cancer Society
New York State Division, Inc.
6725 Lyons St.
East Syracuse, NY 13057
315-437-7025

American Cancer Society
Long Island Division, Inc.
145 Pidgeon Hill Road
Huntington Station, NY 11746
516-385-9100

American Cancer Society
New York City Division, Inc.
19 West 56th St.
New York, NY 10019
212-586-8700

American Caner Society
Queens Division, Inc.
112-25 Queens Blvd.
Forest Hills, NY 11375
718-263-2224

American Cancer Society
Westchester Division, Inc.
30 Glenn St.
White Plains, NY 10603
914-949-4800

NCI Cancer Center
Albert Einstein College of
  Medicine
1300 Morris Park Ave.
Bronx, NY 10461
212-920-4826

NCI Cancer Center
Columbia University
  Comprehensive Cancer
  Center
College of Physicians and
  Surgeons
630 West 168th St.
New York, NY 10032
212-305-6905

NCI Cancer Center
Kaplan Cancer Center
New York University Medical
  Center
462 First Ave.
New York, NY 10016
212-263-6485

NCI Cancer Center
Memorial Sloan-Kettering
  Cancer Center
1275 York Ave.
New York, NY 10021
800-525-2225 or 212-639-2000

NCI Cancer Center
Roswell Park Cancer Center
Elm and Carlton Sts.
Buffalo, NY 14263
716-845-4400

NCI Cancer Center
University of Rochester Cancer
  Center
601 Elmwood Ave.
Rochester, NY 14642
716-275-4911

State Agency
Office of the Aging
Agency Building #2
Empire State Plaza
Albany, NY 12223
518-474-4425

State Agency
Department of Health
Corning Tower Building
Empire State Plaza
Albany, NY 12237
518-474-2011

State Agency
Department of Social Services
Commissioner
40 North Pearl St.
Albany, NY 12243
518-474-9475

State Agency
Insurance Department
Superintendent of Insurance
Empire State Plaza, Agency
 Bldg. #1
Albany, NY 12224
518-474-4550

State Agency
Secretary of State
Department of State Licensing
162 Washington Ave.
Albany, NY 12231
518-474-4750
Medical Conduct 518-474-8357

State Agency
Women's Division
Director
State Capitol
Albany, NY 12224
518-474-3612

PENNSYLVANIA

American Cancer Society
Pennsylvania Division, Inc.
Route 422 and Sipe Ave.
Hershey, PA 17033
717-533-6144

American Cancer Society
Philadelphia Division, Inc.
1422 Chestnut St.
Philadelphia, PA 19102
215-665-2900

NCI Cancer Center
Fox Chase Cancer Center
7701 Burholme Ave.
Philadelphia, PA 19111
215-728-2570

NCI Cancer Center
Pittsburgh Cancer Institute
200 Meyran Ave.
Pittsburgh, PA 15213
800-537-4063

NCI Cancer Center
University of Pennsylvania
 Cancer Center
Penn Tower Hotel, 6th Fl.
3400 Spruce St.
Philadelphia, PA 19104
215-662-6364

State Agency
Department of Aging
Barto Building
231 State St.
Harrisburg, PA 17101
717-783-1550

State Agency
Department of Health
Secretary
802 Health and Welfare
 Building
Harrisburg, PA 17120
717-787-6436

State Agency
Department of Public Welfare
Secretary
333 Health and Welfare
  Building
Harrisburg, PA 17120
717-787-2600

State Agency
Insurance Department
Commissioner
Strawberry Square, 13th Fl.
Harrisburg, PA 17120
717-787-5173

State Agency
Deputy Secretary for Medical
  Assistance
Department of Public Welfare
515 Health and Welfare
  Building
Harrisburg, PA 17120
717-787-1870

State Agency
Professional and Occupational
  Affairs
Department of State
618 Transportation and Safety
  Building
Harrisburg, PA 17120
717-783-7194
Medical Licensing 717-783-7200

State Agency
Commission for Women
Office of the Governor
209 Finance Building
Harrisburg, PA 17120
717-787-8128

Region Three / SOUTHEAST

· ·

FLORIDA
GEORGIA
NORTH CAROLINA
SOUTH CAROLINA
VIRGINIA
WEST VIRGINIA

FLORIDA

American Cancer Society
Florida Division, Inc.
1001 South MacDill Ave.
Tampa, FL 33629
813-253-0541

NCI Cancer Center
Sylvester Comprehensive
 Cancer Center
University of Miami Medical
 School
1475 Northwest 12th Ave.
Miami, FL 33136
305-548-4800

State Agency
Aging and Adult Services
Health and Rehabilitative
 Services
1317 Winewood Blvd., Bldg. 2,
 Rm. 323
Tallahassee, FL 32399
904-488-8922

State Agency
Health Program Office
Health and Rehabilitative
 Services
1317 Winewood Blvd.
Tallahassee, FL 32399
904-487-2705
Board of Medicine
 904-487-7546

State Agency
Insurance Commissioner
State Treasurer
State Capitol
Tallahassee, FL 32399
904-488-3440

State Agency
Deputy Assistant for Medicaid
Health and Rehabilitative
 Services
1317 Winewood Blvd.
Tallahassee, FL 32399
904-488-3560

State Agency
Division of Licensing
Department of State
City Central Building
Tallahassee, FL 32301
904-488-5381
Professional Regulation
904-487-2252

GEORGIA

American Cancer Society
Georgia Division, Inc.
46 Fifth St. NE
Atlanta, GA 30308
404-892-0026

State Agency
Office of Aging
Department of Human
Resources
878 Peachtree St. NE
Atlanta, GA 30309
404-894-2023

State Agency
Public Health Division
Department of Human
Resources
878 Peachtree St. NE
Atlanta, GA 30309
404-894-7505

State Agency
Department of Human
Resources
Commissioner
47 Trinity Ave. SW
Atlanta, GA 30334
404-656-5680

State Agency
Office of Insurance
Comptroller General
2 Martin Luther King Jr. Drive
Atlanta, GA 30334
404-656-2056

State Agency
Department of Medical
Assistance
Commissioner
2 Martin Luther King Jr. Drive
NE
Atlanta, GA 30334
404-656-4479

State Agency
State Examining Board
Office of the Secretary of State
166 Pryor St. SW
Atlanta, GA 30303
404-656-3900
Professional Licensing
404-656-3900

State Agency
Office of the Status for Women
Executive Assistant to the
Governor
245 State Capitol
Atlanta, GA 30334
404-656-1784

NORTH CAROLINA

American Cancer Society
North Carolina Division, Inc.
Suite 221
11 South Boylan Ave.
Raleigh, NC 27603
919-834-8463

NCI Cancer Center
Duke Comprehensive Cancer
Center
P.O. Box 3814
Durham, NC 27710
919-286-5515

NCI Cancer Center
Lineberger Comprehensive
Cancer Center
University of North Carolina
Department of Medicine
Chapel Hill, NC 27599
919-966-4431

State Agency
Assistant Secretary of Aging
Department of Human
Resources
1985 Umstead Dr., Kirby Bldg.
Raleigh, NC 27603
919-733-3983

State Agency
Division of Health Services
Department of Human
Resources
225 North McDowell St.
Raleigh, NC 27603
919-733-3446

State Agency
Department of Human
Resources
Adams Building
101 Blair Drive
Raleigh, NC 27603
919-733-4534

State Agency
Department of Insurance
Commissioner
430 North Salisbury St.
Raleigh, NC 27603
919-733-7343

State Agency
Division of Medical Assistance
Department of Human
Resources
1985 Umstead Drive
Raleigh, NC 27603
919-733-2060
Medical Examiners
919-876-3885

State Agency
Council on Status of Women
Department of Administration
526 North Wilmington St.
Raleigh, NC 27604
919-733-2455

SOUTH CAROLINA

American Cancer Society
South Carolina Division, Inc.
128 Stonemark Lane
Columbia, SC 29210
803-750-1693

State Agency
Commission on Aging
Director
400 Arbor Lake Drive
Columbia, SC 29223
803-735-0210

State Agency
Health and Environmental
Control
Commissioner
2600 Bull St.
Columbia, SC 29201
803-734-4880

State Agency
Department of Social Services
North Complex
1535 Confederate Ave. Ext.
Columbia, SC 29202
803-734-5760

State Agency
Department of Insurance
Chief Insurance Commissioner
1612 Marion St.
Columbia, SC 29201
803-737-6117

State Agency
Health and Human Services
  Finance Commission
Executive Director
P.O. Box 8206
Columbia, SC 29202
803-253-6100
Medical Examiners
  803-734-8901

State Agency
Commission on Women
Chairman
2221 Devine St., Suite 408
Columbia, SC 29205
803-734-9144

VIRGINIA

American Cancer Society
Virginia Division, Inc.
4240 Park Place Court
Glen Allen, VA 23060
804-527-3711

NCI Cancer Center
Massey Cancer Center

Medical College of Virginia
1200 East Broad Street
Richmond, VA 23298
804-786-9641

NCI Cancer Center
University of Virginia Medical
  Center
Primary Care Center, Room
  4520
Box 334, Lee Street
Charlottesville, VA 22908
804-924-2562

State Agency
Department for the Aging
Commissioner
700 East Franklin St., 10th Fl.
Richmond, VA 23219
804-225-2271

State Agency
Department of Health
400 James Madison Building
109 Governor St.
Richmond, VA 23219
804-786-3561

State Agency
Office of Human Resources
Secretary
P.O. Box 1475
Richmond, VA 23212
804-786-7765

State Agency
Department of Insurance
State Corporation Commission
1220 Bank St., 13th Fl.
Richmond, VA 23219
804-786-3603

State Agency
Department of Medical
  Assistance
Suite 1300
600 East Broad St.
Richmond, VA 23219
804-786-7933

State Agency
Department of Commerce
Occupational and Professional
  Licensing
3600 West Broad St., 5th Fl.
Richmond, VA 23220
804-367-8519
Dept. of Health Professions
  804-662-9900

State Agency
Virginia Council on Women
P.O. Box 1475
Richmond VA 23212
804-786-7765

State Agency
Council on the Status of
  Women
Executive Director
8007 Discovery Dr.
Richmond, VA 23288
804-662-9200

WEST VIRGINIA

American Cancer Society
West Virginia Division, Inc.
2428 Kanawha Blvd. East
Charleston, WV 25311
304-344-3611

State Agency
Commissioner on Aging
Executive Director
1710 Kanawha Blvd. East
Charleston, WV 25311
304-348-3317

State Agency
Health and Human Resources
  Department
Building 6, Room B-617
State Capitol Complex
Charleston, WV 25305
304-348-2400
Board of Medicine
  304-348-2921

State Agency
Division of Insurance
Commissioner
2100 Washington St. East
Charleston, WV 25305
304-348-3394

State Agency
Division of Medical Services
Department of Human Services
1900 Washington St. East
Charleston, WV 25305
304-348-8990

State Agency
Women's Commission
Executive Director
WB-9 State Capitol Complex
Charleston, WV 25305
304-348-0070

Region Four / MIDWEST NORTH

ILLINOIS
INDIANA
IOWA
MICHIGAN
MINNESOTA
OHIO
WISCONSIN

ILLINOIS

American Cancer Society
Illinois Division, Inc.
77 East Monroe
Chicago, IL 60603
312-641-6150

NCI Cancer Center
Robert H. Lurie Cancer Center
Room 8250
Olson Pavilion
Chicago, IL 60611
312-908-8400

NCI Cancer Center
Illinois Cancer Center
17th Floor
200 South Michigan Ave.
Chicago, IL 60604
312-986-9980

NCI Cancer Center
University of Chicago
Cancer Research Center
5841 South Maryland Ave.

Chicago, IL 60637
312-702-9200

State Agency
Department on Aging
Director
421 East Capitol
Springfield, IL 62706
217-785-2870

State Agency
Department of Public Health
Director
535 West Jefferson St.
Springfield, IL 62761
217-782-4977

State Agency
Department of Public Aid
Director
316 South Second Ave.
Springfield, IL 62762
217-782-6716

State Agency
Department of Insurance
Director

320 West Washington, 4th Fl.
Springfield, IL 62767
217-782-4515

State Agency
Department of Professional
  Regulation
Director
320 West Washington, 3rd Fl.
Springfield, IL 62786
217-785-0822
Medical Board 217-785-0800

State Agency
Special Assistant for Women
Office of the Governor
100 West Randolph, 16th Fl.
Chicago, IL 60601
312-793-6709

INDIANA

American Cancer Society
Indiana Division, Inc.
8730 Commerce Park Place
Indianapolis, IN 46268
317-872-4432

State Agency
Department of Human Services
P. O. Box 7083
251 N. Illinois St.
Indianapolis, IN 46207
317-232-1139

State Agency
State Board of Health
Commissioner
1330 West Michigan St.
Indianapolis, IN 46206
317-633-8400

State Agency
Department of Public Welfare
Commissioner
100 North Senate Ave., Rm. 701
Indianapolis, IN 46204
317-232-4705

State Agency
Department of Insurance
Commissioner
311 West Washington St., S. 300
Indianapolis, IN 46204
317-232-2386

State Agency
Medicaid Division
Department of Public Welfare
702 State Office Building
Indianapolis, IN 46204
317-232-4324

State Agency
Health Professional Bureau
Executive Director
1 American Square, S. 1020
Indianapolis, IN 46204
317-232-2960

IOWA

American Cancer Society
Iowa Division, Inc.
Suite D
8364 Hickman Road
Des Moines, IA 50325
515-253-0147

State Agency
Department of Elder Affairs
Executive Director
914 Grand, 2nd Fl.
Des Moines, IA 50309
515-281-5187

State Agency
Department of Health
Commissioner
Lucas State Office Building
Des Moines, IA 50319
515-281-5605

State Agency
Department of Human Services
Commissioner
Hoover State Office Building
Des Moines, IA 50319
515-281-5452

State Agency
Insurance Division
Department of Commerce
Lucas State Office Building
Des Moines, IA 50319
515-281-5705

State Agency
Medical Services Bureau
Department of Human Services
Hoover State Office Building
Des Moines, IA 50319
515-281-8621

State Agency
Professional Licensing and
  Regulations
Department of Commerce
1918 SE Hulsizer
Ankeny, IA 50021
515-281-5602
Medical Examiners
  515-281-5171

State Agency
Commission on the Status of
  Women
Administrator
Department of Human Rights
Des Moines, IA 50319
515-281-4461

MICHIGAN

American Cancer Society
Michigan Division, Inc.
1205 East Saginaw Street
Lansing, MI 48906
517-371-2920

NCI Cancer Center
Meyer L. Prentis
  Comprehensive Cancer
  Center of Metropolitan
  Detroit
110 East Warren Ave.
Detroit, MI 48201
313-745-4329

NCI Cancer Center
University of Michigan
Cancer Center
101 Simpson Drive
Ann Arbor, MI 48109
313-936-9583

State Agency
Office of Services to the Aging
Director
P.O. Box 30026
Lansing, MI 48909
517-373-7876

State Agency
Department of Public Health
P.O. Box 30035
3500 North Logan
Lansing, MI 48909
517-335-8024

State Agency
Department of Social Services
P.O. Box 30037
300 South Capitol Ave.
Lansing, MI 48909
517-373-3500

State Agency
Commissioner of Insurance
Licensing and Regulation
  Department
611 West Ottowa, P.O. Box
  30220
Lansing, MI 48909
517-373-9273

State Agency
Medical Services
  Administration
Department of Social Services
P.O. Box 30037
Lansing, MI 48909
517-334-7262

State Agency
Licensing and Regulation
  Department
P.O. Box 30018
611 West Ottawa
Lansing, MI 48909
517-373-1870

State Agency
Women's Commission
Department of Management
  and Budget
P.O. Box 30016
Lansing, MI 48909
517-373-2884

MINNESOTA

American Cancer Society
Minnesota Division, Inc.
3316 West 66th St.
Minneapolis, MN 55435
612-925-2772

NCI Cancer Center
Mayo Comprehensive Cancer
  Center
200 First Street, SW
Rochester, MN 55905
507-284-3413

State Agency
Minnesota Board on Aging
Human Services Building,
  4th Fl.
44 Lafayette Rd.
St. Paul, MN 55155
612-296-2770

State Agency
Department of Health
Commissioner
717 Delaware St., SE
Minneapolis, MN 55440
612-623-5460

State Agency
Department of Human Services
Commissioner
658 Cedar St., 4th Fl.
St. Paul, MN 55155
612-296-2701

State Agency
Commissioner of Insurance
Department of Commerce
Seventh & Robert,
Metro Square Building
St. Paul, MN 55101
612-296-6848

State Agency
Health Care Programs Division
Department of Human Services
444 Lafayette Rd.
St. Paul, MN 55101
612-296-2766

State Agency
Licensing Unit
Department of Commerce
500 Metro Square Building
St. Paul, MN 55101
612-296-6319
Medical Examiners
612-642-0538

State Agency
Commission on the Status of
Women
Executive Director
85 State Office Building
St. Paul, MN 55155
612-296-8590

OHIO

American Cancer Society
Ohio Division, Inc.
5555 Frantz Road
Dublin, OH 43017
614-889-9565

NCI Cancer Center
University Hospitals of
Cleveland
Ireland Cancer Center
2074 Abington Road
Cleveland, OH 44106
216-844-5432

NCI Cancer Center
Ohio State University
Comprehensive Cancer Center
410 West 10th Ave.
Columbus, OH 43210
614-293-8619

State Agency
Commission on Aging
Director
50 West Broad St.
Columbus, OH 43266
614-466-7246

State Agency
Department of Health
Director
246 North High St.
Columbus, OH 43266
614-466-2253
Medical Board 614-466-3934

State Agency
Department of Human Services
Director
30 East Broad St., 32nd Fl.
Columbus, OH 43266
614-466-6282

State Agency
Department of Insurance
Director
2100 Stella Ct.
Columbus, OH 43266
614-481-5728

State Agency
Division of Medical Assistance
Department of Human Services
30 East Broad St., 31st Fl.
Columbus, OH 43266
614-466-2365

State Agency
Women's Division
Bureau of Employment Services
145 South Front St., 6th Fl.
Columbus, OH 43266
614-466-4496

WISCONSIN

American Cancer Society
Wisconsin Division, Inc.
615 North Sherman Ave.
Madison, WI 53704
608-249-0487

NCI Cancer Center
Wisconsin Clinical Cancer
  Center
University of Wisconsin
600 Highland Ave.
Madison, WI 53792
608-263-8090

State Agency
Board on Aging and Long
  Term Care
Department of Administration
122 East Dayton St.
Madison, WI 53702
608-266-8944

State Agency
Division of Health
Health and Social Services
  Dept.
P.O. Box 309
Madison, WI 53701
608-266-1511

State Agency
Health and Social Services
  Dept.
P.O. Box 7850
1 West Wilson
Madison, WI 53707
608-266-3681

State Agency
Commissioner of Insurance
P.O. Box 7873
123 West Washington Ave.
Madison, WI 53707
608-266-3585

State Agency
Division of Health and
  Social Services Dept.
P.O. Box 309
Madison, WI 53701
608-266-1511

State Agency
Regulation and Licensing Dept.
P.O. Box 8935
1400 East Washington
Madison, WI 53708
608-266-8609
Medical Board 608-266-2112

State Agency
Women's Council
Department of Administration
16 North Carroll St., Suite 720
Madison, WI 53702
608-266-2219

Region Five / MIDWEST SOUTH

ALABAMA
ARKANSAS
KENTUCKY
LOUISIANA
MISSISSIPPI
MISSOURI
TENNESSEE

ALABAMA

American Cancer Society
Alabama Division, Inc.
504 Brookwood Blvd.
Homewood, AL 35209
205-879-2242

NCI Cancer Center
University of Alabama at
  Birmingham
Comprehensive Cancer Center
1918 University Blvd., Health
  Bldg.
Birmingham, AL 35294
205-934-6612

State Agency
Commission on Aging
Director
136 Catoma St.
Montgomery, AL 36130
205-242-5743

State Agency
State Health Officer
Department of Public Health
434 Monroe St., Rm. 381
Montgomery, AL 36130
205-242-5052
Medical Examiners
  205-242-4116

State Agency
Department of Human
  Resources
Gordon Persons Building
50 Ripley St.
Montgomery, AL 36130
205-242-1160

State Agency
Insurance Department
Commissioner
64 North Union St., Rm. 504
Montgomery, AL 36130
205-269-3550

State Agency
Medicaid Agency
Commissioner
2500 Fairlane Drive
Montgomery, AL 36130
205-277-2710

ARKANSAS

American Cancer Society
Arkansas Division, Inc.
901 North University
Little Rock, AR 72207
501-664-3480

State Agency
Aging and Adult Services
1428 Donaghey Bldg.
Seventh & Main St.
Little Rock, AR 72201
501-682-2441

State Agency
Department of Health
Director
4815 West Markham St.
Little Rock, AR 72205
501-661-2111
Medical Board 508-578-2448

State Agency
Department of Human Services
Director
P.O. Box 1437, Slot 316
Little Rock, AR 72203
501-682-8650

State Agency
Insurance Department
Commissioner

400 University Tower Bldg.
Little Rock, AR 72204
501-371-1325

State Agency
Economic & Medical Services
Division
Department of Human Services
P.O. Box 1437, Slot 316
Little Rock, AR 72203
501-682-8375

KENTUCKY

American Cancer Society
Kentucky Division, Inc.
701 West Muhammad Ali Blvd.
Louisville, KY 40201
502-584-6782

State Agency
Aging Services Division
Department for Social Services
275 East Main St.
Frankfort, KY 40601
502-564-6930

State Agency
Department for Health Services
Cabinet for Human Resources
275 East Main St.
Frankfort, KY 40601
502-564-3970

State Agency
Cabinet for Human Resources
Secretary
275 East Main St.
Frankfort, KY 40601
502-564-7130

State Agency
Department of Insurance
Public Protection & Reg.
 Cabinet
229 West Main St.
Frankfort, KY 40601
502-564-6027

State Agency
Department for Medicaid
 Services
Cabinet for Human Resources
275 East Main St.
Frankfort, KY 40601
502-564-4321

State Agency
Occupations & Professions
 Division
Department of Administration
P.O. Box 456, Capitol Annex
Frankfort, KY 40601
502-564-3296
Medical Licensure 502-896-1516

State Agency
Commission on Women
Executive Director
614A Shelby St.
Frankfort, KY 40601
502-564-6643

LOUISIANA

American Cancer Society
Louisiana Division, Inc.
Fidelity Homestead Bldg.
837 Gravier St., Suite 700
New Orleans, LA 70112
504-523-4188

State Agency
Office of Elderly Affairs
Office of the Governor
P.O. Box 80374
Baton Rouge, LA 70898
504-925-1700

State Agency
Department of Health &
 Hospitals
Secretary
325 Loyola Ave.
New Orleans, LA 70112
504-568-5050

State Agency
Department of Insurance
Commissioner
P.O. Box 94214
Baton Rouge, LA 70804
504-342-5322

State Agency
Medicaid Eligibility Office
Health & Human Resources
 Department
P.O. Box 9465
Baton Rouge, LA 70804
504-342-3950

State Agency
Office of Licensing &
 Regulation
Health & Human Resources
 Department
P.O. Box 3767
Baton Rouge, LA 70821
504-342-6447
Medical Examiners
 504-524-6763

State Agency
Office of Women's Services
Division of Administration
P.O. Box 94095
Baton Rouge, LA 70806
504-342-2715

MISSISSIPPI

American Cancer Society
Mississippi Division, Inc.
Lakeover Office Park
1380 Livingston Lane
Jackson, MS 39213
601-362-8874

State Agency
Council on Aging
Department of Human
  Development
301 West Pearl St.
Jackson, MS 39203
601-354-6590

State Agency
State Health Officer
Department of Health
2423 North State St.
Jackson, MS 39216
601-354-6646
Medical Licensure
  601-354-6645

State Agency
Department of Insurance
Commissioner
1804 Sillers Bldg.
Jackson, MS 39201
601-359-3569

State Agency
Division of Medicaid
Office of the Governor
239 North Lamar St., #8011
Jackson, MS 39202
601-359-6050

MISSOURI

American Cancer Society
Missouri Division, Inc.
3322 American Ave.
Jefferson City, MO 65109
314-893-4800

State Agency
Division on Aging
Department of Social Services
P.O. Box 1337
Jefferson City, MO 65102
314-751-3082

State Agency
Department of Health
Director
P.O. Box 570
Jefferson City, MO 65102
314-751-6001

State Agency
Department of Social Services
Broadway Building
P.O. Box 1527
Jefferson City, MO 65102
314-751-4815

State Agency
Division of Insurance
Department of Economic
  Development

Truman Bldg., Box 690
Jefferson City, MO 65102
314-751-2451

State Agency
Division of Medical Services
Department of Social Services
308 East High, Box 6500
Jefferson City, MO 65103
314-751-3425

State Agency
Professional Registration
  Division
Department of Economic
  Development
P.O. Box 1335
Jefferson City, MO 65102
314-751-2334
Medical Licensing 314-751-2334

State Agency
Council on Women's Economic
  Development & Training
Truman Bldg., Box 1157
Jefferson City, MO 65102
314-751-0810

TENNESSEE

American Cancer Society
Tennessee Division, Inc.
1315 Eighth Ave. South
Nashville, TN 37203
615-255-1227

NCI Cancer Center
Drew-Meharry-Morehouse
  Consortium Cancer Center

1005 D. B. Todd Blvd.
Nashville, TN 37208
615-327-6927

NCI Cancer Center
St. Jude Children's Research
  Hospital
332 North Lauderdale St.
Memphis, TN 38101
901-522-0306

State Agency
Commission on Aging
715 Tennessee Bldg.
535 Church St.
Nashville, TN 37219
615-741-2056

State Agency
Department of Health &
  Environment
Commissioner
344 Cordell Hull Bldg.
Nashville, TN 37219
615-741-3111

State Agency
Department of Human Services
Commissioner
111 Seventh Ave. N., 12th Fl.
Nashville, TN 37219
615-741-3241

State Agency
Department of Commerce &
  Insurance
Suite 1400
1808 West End Rd.
Nashville, TN 37219
615-741-2241

State Agency
Medicaid Administration
Department of Health &
  Environment
Terra Bldg., 5th Fl.
Nashville, TN 37219
615-741-0213

State Agency
Regulatory Boards
Department of Commerce &
  Insurance
1808 West End Bldg., 9th Fl.
Nashville, TN 37219
615-741-3449
Medical Board 615-741-3111

Region Six / CENTRAL NORTH

MONTANA
NEBRASKA
NORTH DAKOTA
SOUTH DAKOTA
WYOMING

MONTANA

American Cancer Society
Montana Division, Inc.
17 North 26th
Billings, MT 59101
406-252-7111

State Agency
Aging Unit Contracts Bureau
Department of Social &
    Rehabilitation Services
111 Sanders St.
Helena, MT 59601
406-444-5650

State Agency
Health Services Division
Health & Environmental
    Sciences
Capitol Station
Helena, MT 59620
406-444-2037

State Agency
Department of Social &
    Rehabilitation Services
111 Sanders St.
Helena, MT 59601
406-444-5622

State Agency
Insurance Division
Office of State Auditor
Mitchell Building
Helena, MT 59620
406-444-2996

State Agency
Economic Assistance Division
Social & Rehabilitation Services
111 Sanders St.
Helena, MT 59601
406-444-4540

State Agency
Professional & Occupational
    Licensing
Department of Commerce
1424 Ninth Ave.
Helena, MT 59620
406-444-3768
Medical Examiner
    406-444-4370

State Agency
Council on Women &
  Employment
Governor's Office
State Capitol
Helena, MT 59620
406-444-3111

NEBRASKA

American Cancer Society
Nebraska Division, Inc.
8502 West Center Road
Omaha, NE 68124
402-393-5800

NCI Cancer Center
Eppley Institute
University of Nebraska Medical
  Center
600 South 42nd Street
Omaha, NE 68198
402-559-4000

State Agency
Department on Aging
P.O. Box 95044
301 Centennial Mall S.
Lincoln, NE 68509
402-471-2306

State Agency
Department of Health
P.O. Box 95007
301 Centennial Mall S.
Lincoln, NE 68509
402-471-2133
Board of Medical Examiners
  402-471-2133

State Agency
Department of Insurance
The Terminal Building
941 O St., Suite 400
Lincoln, NE 68508
402-471-2201

State Agency
Medical Services Administrator
Department of Social Services
P.O. Box 95026
Lincoln, NE 68509
402-471-3121

State Agency
Bureau of Examining Board
Department of Health
P.O. Box 95007
Lincoln, NE 68509
402-471-2115

State Agency
Commission on Status of
  Women
P.O. Box 94985
301 Centennial Mall S.
Lincoln, NE 68509
402-471-2039

NORTH DAKOTA

American Cancer Society
North Dakota Division, Inc.
123 Roberts Street
Fargo, ND 58102
701-232-1385

State Agency
Aging Services
Department of Human Services
State Capital, Judicial Wing
Bismarck, ND 58505
701-224-2577

State Agency
Department of Health
State Health Officer
600 East Blvd., State Capitol
Bismarck, ND 58505
701-224-2372

State Agency
Department of Human Services
State Capitol, Judicial Wing
600 East Blvd.
Bismarck, ND 58505
701-224-2310

State Agency
Insurance Department
State Capitol, 5th Fl.
600 E. Blvd.
Bismarck, ND 58505
701-224-2440

State Agency
Medical Services Division
Department of Human Services
600 East Blvd., State Capitol
Bismarck, ND 58505
701-224-2321

State Agency
Occupational & Professional
  Licensing
Secretary of State
State Capitol, 1st Fl.
600 East Blvd.
Bismarck, ND 58505
701-224-2900
Medical Examiners
  701-223-9485

State Agency
Commission on Status of
  Women
Department of Human Services
600 East Blvd., Judicial Wing
Bismarck, ND 58505
701-224-2970

SOUTH DAKOTA

American Cancer Society
South Dakota Division, Inc.
4101 Carnegie Place
Sioux Falls, SD 57106
605-361-8277

State Agency
Division of Adult Services &
  Aging
Department of Social Services
Kneip Bldg.
Pierre, SD 57501
605-773-3656

State Agency
Department of Health
Secretary
Foss Building
Pierre, SD 57501
605-773-3361

State Agency
Department of Human Services
Secretary
Kneip Building
Pierre, SD 57501
605-773-3165

State Agency
Division of Insurance
Commerce & Regulations
Department
910 East Sioux, State Capitol
Pierre, SD 57501
605-773-3563

State Agency
Office of Medical Services
Department of Social Services
Kneip Building
Pierre, SD 57501
605-773-3495

State Agency
Professional & Occupational
Licensing
Commerce & Regulations
Department
910 East Sioux Ave.
Pierre, SD 57501
605-773-3177
Board of Medical Examiners
605-336-1965

WYOMING

American Cancer Society
Wyoming Division
2222 House Ave.
Cheyenne, WY 82001
307-638-3331

State Agency
Commission on Aging
Director
Hathaway Building, Rm. 139
Cheyenne, WY 82002
307-777-7986

State Agency
Health & Medical Services
Division.

Health & Social Services
Department
Hathaway Building
Cheyenne, WY 82002
307-777-7121

State Agency
Human Resources Coordinator
State Planning Coordinator's
Office
Office of the Governor
Cheyenne, WY 82002
307-777-7574

State Agency
Insurance Department
Commissioner
Herschler Building
Cheyenne, WY 82002
307-777-7401

State Agency
Medical Assistance
Health & Medical Services
Division
Hathaway Building
Cheyenne, WY 82002
307-777-7531

State Agency
Department of Commerce
Occupational & Professional
Licensing
Barrett Building
Cheyenne, WY 82002
307-777-6303
Board of Medical Examiners
307-777-6463

State Agency
Commission for Women
Department of Labor &
Statistics
Herschler Building
Cheyenne, WY 82002
307-777-7349

Region Seven / CENTRAL SOUTH
· ·

ARIZONA
COLORADO
KANSAS
NEW MEXICO
OKLAHOMA
TEXAS
UTAH

ARIZONA

American Cancer Society
Arizona Division, Inc.
2929 East Thomas Road
Phoenix, AZ 85016
602-224-0524

NCI Cancer Center
University of Arizona
Cancer Center
1501 North Campbell Ave.
Tucson, AZ 85724
602-626-6372

State Agency
Division of Aging, Family &
Children's Services
1400 West Washington
Phoenix, AZ 85007
602-255-4446

State Agency
Department of Health Services
Room 407
1740 West Adams St.

Phoenix, AZ 85007
602-542-1024
Medical Examiners
602-255-3751

State Agency
Department of Economic
Security
Director
1717 West Jefferson
Phoenix, AZ 85007
602-542-5678

State Agency
Department of Insurance
Room 200
3030 North Third St.
Phoenix, AZ 85012
602-255-5400

State Agency
Arizona Health Care Cost
Containment System
801 East Jefferson
Phoenix, AZ 85034
602-234-3655

State Agency
Department of Economic
  Security
Director
1717 West Jefferson
Phoenix, AZ 85007
602-542-5678

COLORADO

American Cancer Society
Colorado Division, Inc.
2255 South Oneida
Denver, CO 80224
303-758-2030

NCI Cancer Center
University of Colorado Cancer
  Center
University of Colorado Health
  Sciences Center
4200 East 9th Ave., Box B188
Denver, CO 80262
303-270-3007

State Agency
Aging & Adult Services
  Division
Department of Social Services
1575 Sherman St., 10th Fl.
Denver, CO 80203
303-866-2580

State Agency
Department of Health
Executive Director
4210 East 11th Ave.
Denver, CO 80220
303-331-4600

State Agency
Human Services Division
Department of Social Services
1575 Sherman St.
Denver, CO 80203
303-866-3448

State Agency
Division of Insurance
Department of Regulatory
  Agencies
303 West Colfax Ave., 5th Fl.
Denver, CO 80204
303-866-3201

State Agency
Division of Medical Assistance
Department of Social Services
1757 Sherman St., Rm. 617
Denver, CO 80203
303-866-5901

State Agency
Department of Regulatory
  Agencies
Executive Director
1525 Sherman St., Rm. 110
Denver, CO 80203
303-866-3304
Medical Examiners
  303-894-7690

KANSAS

American Cancer Society
Kansas Division, Inc.
1315 SW Arrowhead Rd.
Topeka, KS 66604
913-273-4114

State Agency
Department of Aging
Secretary, 122S
Docking State Office Bldg.
Topeka, KS 66612
913-296-4986

State Agency
Division of Health
Department of Health &
Environment
Landon St. Office Bldg.,
Rm. 1052
Topeka, KS 66620
913-296-1343
State Board 913-296-7413

State Agency
Department of Social &
Rehabilitative Services
Secretary
State Office Bldg., 6th Fl.
Topeka, KS 66612
913-296-3271

State Agency
Insurance Department
Secretary
420 SW Ninth St.
Topeka, KS 66612
913-296-3071

State Agency
Division of Medical Programs
Department of Social &
Rehabilitative Services
State Office Bldg., 6th Fl.
Topeka, KS 66612
913-296-3981

NEW MEXICO

American Cancer Society
New Mexico Division, Inc.
5800 Lomas Blvd., NE
Albuquerque, NM 87110
505-260-2105

State Agency
State Agency on Aging
Director
224 East Palace Ave., 4th Fl.
Santa Fe, NM 87501
505-827-7640

State Agency
Department of Health &
Environment
Deputy Secretary
1190 St. Francis Dr., Rm N4100
Santa Fe, NM 87503
505-984-2000

State Agency
Department of Human Services
Secretary
PERA Building
Santa Fe, NM 87503
505-827-4065

State Agency
State Insurance Board Division
State Corporation Commission
PERA Building, Rm. 428
Santa FE, NM 87503
505-827-4297

State Agency
Medical Assistance Division
Department of Human Services
PERA Building

Santa Fe, NM 87503
505-827-4315

State Agency
Department of Regulation &
  Licensing
Superintendent
Bataan Memorial Bldg.,
  Rm. 133
Santa Fe, NM 87503
505-827-6318
Medical Board 505-827-4200

State Agency
Commission on the Status of
  Women
Executive Director
5006 Cooper NE
Albuquerque, NM 87108
505-841-4665

OKLAHOMA

American Cancer Society
Oklahoma Division, Inc.
Suite 136
3000 United Founders Blvd.
Oklahoma City, OK 73112

State Agency
Department of Human Services
Director
P.O. Box 25352
Oklahoma City, OK 73125
405-521-3646

State Agency
Department of Health
P.O. Box 53551
1000 NE Tenth
Oklahoma City, OK 73152

405-271-4200
State Board of Licensing
405-848-2189

State Agency
Social Services
Secretary
212 State Capitol
Oklahoma City, OK 73105
405-521-2342

State Agency
Insurance Department
Commissioner
408 Will Rogers Bldg.
Oklahoma City, OK 73105
405-521-2828

State Agency
Intergovernmental Affairs
Department for Women
440 South Houston St.,
  Suite 304
Tulsa, OK 74127
918-581-2801

TEXAS

American Cancer Society
Texas Division Inc.
2433 Ridgepoint Drive
Austin, TX 78754
512-928-2262

NCI Cancer Center
Institute for Cancer Research
  and Care
4450 Medical Drive
San Antonio, TX 78229
512-616-5580

NCI Cancer Center
The University of Texas
M. D. Anderson Cancer Center
1515 Holcombe Blvd.
Houston, TX 77030
713-792-3245

State Agency
Department on Aging
Box 12786
Capitol Station
Austin, TX 78711
512-444-2727

State Agency
Department of Health
Commissioner
1100 West 49th St.
Austin, TX 78756
512-458-7375
Medical Examiner
  512-452-1078

State Agency
Department of Human Services
Commissioner
P.O. Box 2960
Austin, TX 78769
512-450-3030

State Agency
Board of Insurance
Commissioner
1100 San Jacinto Blvd.
Austin, TX 78701
512-463-6464

State Agency
Commission on Women
Office of the Governor
Box 12428, Capitol Station
Austin, TX 78711
512-463-1782

UTAH

American Cancer Society
Utah Division, Inc.
610 East South Temple
Salt Lake City, UT 84102
801-322-0431

NCI Cancer Center
Utah Regional Cancer Center
University of Utah Medical
  Center
50 North Medical Drive,
  Rm. 2C10
Salt Lake City, UT 84132
801-581-5052

State Agency
Division of Aging
Department of Social Services
120 North 200 W., Rm. 401
Salt Lake City, UT 84103
801-538-3910

State Agency
Department of Health
P.O. Box 2500
288 North 1460 W.
Salt Lake City, UT 84116
801-538-6111

State Agency
Department of Social Services
Executive Director
120 North 200 W.
Salt Lake City, UT 84103
801-538-3998

State Agency
Department of Insurance
Commissioner
160 East 300 S.

Salt Lake City, UT 84111
801-530-6400

State Agency
Division of Health Care
  Financing
Department of Health
288 North 1460, W., Box 16580
Salt Lake City, UT 84116
801-538-6151

State Agency
Division of Occupational &
  Professional Licensing
Box 45802
160 East 300 S.
Salt Lake City, UT 84111
801-530-6620
Medical Licensing
  801-530-6626

Region Eight / PACIFIC
. . . .

ALASKA
CALIFORNIA
HAWAII
IDAHO
NEVADA
OREGON
WASHINGTON

ALASKA

American Cancer Society
Alaska Division, Inc.
Suite 204
406 West Fireweed Lane
Anchorage, AK 99503
907-277-8696

State Agency
Older Alaskans Commission
Department of Administration
P.O. Box C
Juneau, AK 99811
907-465-3250

State Agency
Department of Health & Social
  Services
Commissioner
P.O. Box H-01
Juneau, AK 99811
907-465-3030

State Agency
Division of Insurance
Commerce & Economic
  Development
P.O. Box D
Juneau, AK 99811
907-465-2515

State Agency
Division of Medical Assistance
Health & Social Services
  Department
P.O. Box H-07
Juneau, AK 99811
907-465-3355

State Agency
Occupational Licensing
  Division
Commerce & Economic
  Development
P.O. Box D
Juneau, AK 99811
907-465-2534
Medical Board 907-561-2878

State Agency
Alaska Women's Commission
Office of the Governor
3601 C St., Suite 742
Anchorage, AK 99503
907-561-4227

CALIFORNIA

American Cancer Society
California Division, Inc.
1710 Webster St.
Oakland, CA 94612
510-893-7900

NCI Cancer Center
City of Hope National Medical
   Center
Beckman Research Institute
1500 East Duarte Road
Duarte, CA 91010
818-359-8111

NCI Cancer Center
Jonsson Comprehensive Cancer
   Center
University of California at Los
   Angeles
200 Medical Plaza
Los Angeles, CA 90027
213-206-0278

NCI Cancer Center
The Kenneth Norris Jr.
   Comprehensive Cancer
   Center, University of
   Southern California
1441 Eastlake Ave.
Los Angeles, CA 90033
213-226-2370

NCI Cancer Center
University of California at San
   Diego Cancer Center
225 Dickinson St.
San Diego, CA 92103
619-543-6178

State Agency
Department of Aging
Director
1600 K St.
Sacramento, CA 95814
916-322-5290

State Agency
Department of Health Services
Director
714 P St., Rm. 1253
Sacramento, CA 95814
916-445-1248

State Agency
Health & Welfare Agency
Secretary
1600 Ninth St., Rm. 460
Sacramento, CA 95814
916-445-1722

State Agency
Department of Insurance
Commissioner
600 South Commonwealth Ave.
Los Angeles, CA 90005
213-736-2551

State Agency
Medi-Cal Operations Division
Department of Health Services
714 P St., Rm. 1540
Sacramento, CA 95814
916-324-2681

State Agency
Department of Consumer
 Affairs
Director
1020 N St., Rm. 516
Sacramento, CA 95814
916-445-4465
Medical Board 916-920-6343

HAWAII

American Cancer Society
Hawaii/Pacific Division, Inc.
Community Services Center
 Bldg.
200 North Vineyard Blvd.
Honolulu, HI 96817
808-531-1662

State Agency
Executive Office of Aging
Office of the Governor
335 Merchant St., Rm. 241
Honolulu, HI 96813
808-548-2593

State Agency
Department of Health
Director
1250 Punchbowl St.
Honolulu, HI 96813
808-548-6505

State Agency
Department of Human Services
Director
1390 Miller St.
Honolulu, HI 96813
808-548-6260

State Agency
Division of Insurance
Department of Commerce &
 Consumer Affairs
1010 Richards St.
Honolulu, HI 96813
808-548-6522

State Agency
Department of Commerce &
 Consumer Affairs
Director
1010 Richards St.
Honolulu, HI 96813
808-548-7505
Medical Examiners
 808-548-4392

State Agency
Commission on the Status of
 Women
Department of Human Services
335 Merchant St., Rm. 253
Honolulu, HI 96813
808-548-4199

State Agency
Health Care Administrative
 Division
Department of Human Services
820 Mililani, Rm. 817
Honolulu, HI 96813
808-548-6584

IDAHO

American Cancer Society
Idaho Division, Inc.
2676 Vista Ave.
Boise, ID 83705
208-343-4609

State Agency
Office on Aging
Director
Statehouse
Boise, ID 83720
208-334-3833

State Agency
Department of Health and
  Welfare
Director
Statehouse
Boise, ID 83720
208-334-5700

State Agency
Department of Insurance
Director
500 South 10th St.
Boise, ID 83720
208-334-2250

State Agency
Division of Welfare
Department of Health &
  Welfare
450 West State St.
Boise, ID 83720
208-334-5747

State Agency
Occupational Licenses
Self-Governing Agencies
2417 Bank Dr., #312
Boise, ID 83705
208-334-3233
Board of Medicine
  208-334-2822

State Agency
Commission on Women's
  Progress
Director

P.O. Box 4989
Pocatello, ID 84201
208-234-0020

NEVADA

American Cancer Society
Nevada Division, Inc.
1325 East Harmon
Las Vegas, NV 89119
702-798-6857

State Agency
Division for Aging Services
Department of Human
  Resources
505 East King St.
Carson City, NV 89710
702-885-4210

State Agency
Health Division
Department of Human
  Resources
505 East King St.
Carson City, NV 89710
702-885-4740
Medical Examiners
  702-329-2559 or 486-6244

State Agency
Department of Human
  Resources
Director
505 East King St.
Carson City, NV 89710
702-885-4400

State Agency
Insurance Division
Department of Commerce
201 South Fall St.
Carson City, NV 89701
702-885-4270

State Agency
Medicaid Division
Department of Human
  Resources
2527 North Carson St.
Carson City, NV 89710
702-885-4698

OREGON

American Cancer Society
Oregon Division, Inc.
330 SW Curry
Portland, OR 97201
503-295-6422

State Agency
Senior Services Division
Department of Human
  Resources
313 Public Service Building
Salem, OR 97310
503-378-4728

State Agency
Health Division
Department of Human
  Resources
1400 SW Fifth Ave.
Portland, OR 97201
503-229-5032

State Agency
Department of Human
  Resources
Director
318 Public Service Building
Salem, OR 97310
503-378-3034

State Agency
Department of Insurance &
  Finance
Director
21 Labor & Industries Building
Salem, OR 97310
503-378-4120
Medical Examiners
  503-229-5770

State Agency
Adult Family Services Division
Department of Human
  Resources
203 Public Service Building
Salem, OR 97310
503-378-2263

State Agency
Commission for Women
Executive Director
695 Summer St., NE
Salem, OR 97310
503-378-2780

WASHINGTON

American Cancer Society
Washington Division, Inc.
2120 First Avenue N.
Seattle, WA 98109
206-283-1152

NCI Cancer Center
Fred Hutchinson Cancer
  Research Center
1124 Columbia St.
Seattle, WA 98104
206-467-4675

State Agency
Aging & Adult Services
  Administration
Department of Social & Health
  Services
Office Building #2, M/S:
  OB-44A
Olympia, WA 98504
206-586-3768

State Agency
Department of Health
M/S:EY-12
1300 Quince
Olympia, WA 98504
206-586-5846
Medical Board 206-753-5871

State Agency
Department of Social & Health
  Services
M/S: OB-44
Office Building #2
Olympia, WA 98504
206-753-3395

State Agency
Office of the Insurance
  Commissioner
M/S:AQ-21
Insurance Building
Olympia, WA 98504
206-753-7301

State Agency
Division of Medical Assistance
Department of Social & Health
  Services
Town Square Building B, M/S:
  HB-41
Olympia, WA 98504
206-753-1777

State Agency
Department of Licensing
M/S: PB-01
Highway–Licenses Building
Olympia, WA 98504
206-753-2241

SECTION TWO

National Organizations and Associations

A listing of national organizations and associations equipped to provide you with information of all types relating to breast cancer. Some have 800 numbers or hotlines so that you can receive information quickly.

American Association of Retired Persons (AARP)
Health Care Campaign
601 E Street, N.W.
Washington, DC 20049
202-434-3828
Membership communications office has a number of pamphlets and brochures on health care and health-related issues important to older Americans.

American Cancer Society
National Headquarters
1599 Clifton Road, N.E.
Atlanta, GA 30329
404-320-3333
1-800-227-2345 Cancer
Response System
Brochures, pamphlets, information relating to cancer; 3,000 chapters nationwide to give local guidance on hospitals, specialists, and treatments.

American Institute for Cancer Research
1759 R Street, N.W.
Washington, DC 20009
1-800-834-8114
Has newsletter and other publications on nutrition and cancer risks. Publishes a booklet on breast lumps and breast cancer.

American Medical Association
P.O. Box 109050
Chicago, IL 60610
1-800-621-8335 order
department
Organization monitoring the medical industry and its related fields.

American Medical Record Association
875 North Michigan Avenue,
Suite 1850
Chicago, IL 60611
312-787-2672
Can give assistance if you have a problem obtaining your medical records.

211

Americans for Medical Progress
Educational Foundation
Crystal Square Three
1735 Jefferson Davis Highway
Arlington, VA 22202
703-486-1411
Provides grassroots support for medical research.

Association of Academic Health Centers
1400 16th Street, NW, Suite 410
Washington, DC 20036
202-265-9600
Involved with total health education; sponsors task forces; develops research and education programs. Will send a list of over 100 members and their associated medical schools ($13).

Breast Cancer Advisory Center
11426 Rockville Pike, Suite 406
Rockville, MD 20850
301-984-1040
Medical service group for women with breast cancer; makes referrals, gives lectures, and provides information.

Cancer Care
National Cancer Care
  Foundation
1180 Avenue of the Americas
New York, NY 10036
212-221-3300 or 800-367-4357
Oldest voluntary cancer support agency. Provides financial advice, professional counseling, transportation, and guidance for cancer patients and their families.

Cancer Information Service
National Cancer Institute
9000 Rockville Pike
Bethesada, MD 20892
800-422-6237 Alaska
  800-638-6070
Hawaii 808-524-1234
National network of information, publications, treatment centers, doctors, programs, research relating to cancer. Can direct you to local CIS.

Cancer Research Council
4853 Cordell Avenue, Suite 11
Bethesda, MD 20814
301-654-7933
Has information on new experimental medical treatments for cancer.

Coalition for the Medical Rights of Women
1638-B Haight Street
San Francisco, CA 94117
415-621-8030
Organization concerned with health care for women; increases public awareness, education, policies; clearinghouse library on women's health issues.

Health Facts
Center for Medical Consumers
  and Health Care Information
237 Thompson Street
New York, NY 10012
212-674-7105
Has reports on risks associated with drugs and other medical treatments.

International Association of Cancer Victors and Friends
Number 110
7740 West Manchester Avenue
Playa Del Ray, CA 90293
213-822-5032
Supports cancer research, provides information on treatments, and works with patients and area service organizations.

Make Today Count
101½ South Union Street
Alexandria, VA 22314
703-548-9674
Services cancer patients and immediate families, has educational programs, films, tapes; can direct you to appropriate community services.

National Alliance of Breast Cancer Organizations
1180 Avenue of Americas
New York, NY 10036
212-719-0154
Follows latest research and treatments; has resource list, special mailings, and newsletter. Prefers written inquiries.

National Cancer Institute
Office of Cancer Communications
9000 Rockville Pike
Building 31, Room 10A18
Bethesda, MD 20892
301-496-5583 800-422-6237
Physician Data Query
Information specialist will guide you to specific cancer treatments and clinical trials and will send you a database printout.

National Council Against Health Fraud
Consumer Health Information Research Institute
3521 Broadway
Kansas City, MO 64111
800-821-6671
Will verify alternative cancer treatments; can assist you if you suspect questionable health practices.

National Health Information Center
P.O. Box 1133
Washington, DC 20013
301-565-4167 800-336-4979
A clearinghouse for written materials on health and health related information. Can direct you to other organizations and services.

National Institutes of Health
Office of Medical Applications
9000 Rockville Pike
Bethesda, MD 20892
301-496-2433
NIH will provide a statement on mastectomy vs. lumpectomy, adjuvant therapy, and early stage breast cancer.

National Lymphedema Network (NLN)
2211 Post Street, Suite 404
San Francisco, CA 94115
800-541-3259
A nonprofit resource organization providing support and information about lymphedema, its treatment and prevention.

National Second Opinion Program
52 Vanderbilt Avenue, Room 1503
New York, NY 10017
212-370-7821 in New York
800-631-1220
1-800-522-0036
Serves individuals seeking medical assistance on second opinion consultations; works on health care cost containment.

National Rural Health Association
301 East Armour Blvd., Suite 420
Kansas City, MO 64111
816-756-3140
Includes all varieties of professionals involved in rural health care problems; supplies current information to rural providers and acts as liaison to facilities.

National Self-Help Clearing House
33 West 42nd Street
New York, NY 10036
212-642-2944
Lists information on cancer organizations, support groups, community health services, rehabilitation. Send self-addressed stamped envelope.

National Women's Health Network
1325 G Street, NW
Washington, DC 20005
202-347-1140
Monitors federal health policy; has clearinghouse of national resources on all aspects of women's health care and related issues; provides information and referrals.

Public Citizen Health Research Group
2000 P Street, NW, Sixth Fl.
Washington, DC 20036
202-833-3000
Works on issues of health care delivery; petitions federal agencies on consumers behalf; monitors the enforcement of health legislation; lists questionable doctors.

Reach to Recovery
c/o American Cancer Society
1599 Clifton Road, NE
Atlanta, GA 30329
404-320-3333
One-on-one help for women who have had breast cancer; pre- and post-operative information and support. Variety of breast information.

SHARE
817 Broadway, Sixth Fl.
New York, NY 10003
212-260-0580
Self-help organization for women with breast cancer; offers support groups; has library on all forms of treatment information.

The Chemotherapy Foundation
183 Madison Avenue, Suite 403
New York, NY 10016
212-213-9292
Will provide a pamphlet on the positive and negative effects of chemotherapy and another pamphlet on breast cancer.

The Susan G. Komen Foundation
5005 LBJ Freeway, Suite 730
Dallas, TX 75244
800-462-9273 or 214-450-1777
Supports research on cancer; promotes public awareness and early detection; sponsors educational programs. Has books and information on breast cancer.

The Y-ME National Organization of Breast Cancer Information and Support
18220 Harwood Avenue
Homewood, IL 60430
708-799-8228 9-5 Central Time
800-221-2141 24 hr. 7 day
Provides information and support for women with breast cancer; can connect you with other breast cancer patients.

The YWCA Encore Program
National Headquarters
726 Broadway
New York, NY 10003
212-614-2827
Provides support and rehabilitation for women who have had breast cancer. Contact them for the program nearest you.

SECTION THREE

Organizations and Government Agencies with Information on Financial Assistance, Insurance, and Public Advocacy

Lists of national organizations, associations, and government agencies that can help with the business aspects of breast cancer. These include information on insurance, financial assistance, verification of facilities, retrieval of medical records, and public advocacy groups.

Agency for Health Care Policy and Research
Publications Clearinghouse
P.O. Box 8547
Silver Spring, MD 20907
800-358-9295 301-227-8168
Information on health insurance, plans, terms, and services. Offers worksheet and booklet on health insurance choices. Wide range of information.

American Association of Preferred Provider Organizations
111 East Wacker Drive, Suite 600
Chicago, IL 60601
312-644-6610
Members are preferred provider organizations and individuals associated with the PPO industry.

American Association of Retired Persons
AARP Fulfillment
1909 K Street, NW
Washington, DC 20036
202-434-3828
Offers information on Medicare and insurance through their Health Advocacy Program.

American Health Decisions
Department P
1200 Larimer Street, Campus Box 133
Denver, CO 80224
303-534-3000
An organization that will put you in touch with grass-roots groups that discuss health-care issues and lobby for change in the health industry.

American Managed Care and Review Association
1227 25th Street, NW, #610
Washington, DC 20037
202-778-0506
Members include health maintenance organizations, preferred provider organizations, and other groups offering managed care.

American Public Health Association
1015 15th Street, NW, #300
Washington, DC 20005
202-789-5600
Members include health-care professionals interested in health care and education. Produces data on female workers in public health and their health status.

Association of Community Cancer Centers
11620 Nebel Street, #201
Rockville, MD 20852
301-984-9496
Membership includes community hospitals involved in providing cancer care. Encourages clinical research. Offers information and help on insurance coverage and costs relating to cancer drugs and treatments.

**CAN ACT
Cancer Patients Action Alliance**
26 College Place
Brooklyn, NY 11201
718-260-8184
Cancer patient organization involved in legislation to increase

access to drugs for all cancer patients. Has updates on current changes.

Command Trust Network, Inc.
The Breast Implant
Information Network
P.O. Box 17082
Covington, KY 41017
606-331-0055 213-556-1738
Provides information and assistance regarding breast implants. Newsletter and other written materials.

Consumer Health Information Research Institute
3521 Broadway
Kansas City, MO 64111
800-821-6671
Investigates information on alternative cancer treatments and potential health fraud issues.

Food and Drug Administration
Breast Implant Information
5600 Fishers Lane
Rockville, MD 20857
800-532-4440 301-443-3170
Conducts research on the quality and safety of the medical industry. Accepts inquiries and complaints on breast implants.

Group Health Association of America
1129 20th Street, NW, Suite 600
Washington, DC 20036
202-778-3200
Members include health maintenance organizations and other group medical practices that take prepayment.

**Health Care Financing
Administration**
Department of Health and
  Human Services
200 Independence Avenue, SW
Washington, DC 20201
202-690-6726
*Administers Medicare and
Medicaid (a health insurance
program for persons judged unable
to pay for health services).*

**Health Care Financing
Administration**
Survey and Certification
6325 Security Boulevard
Baltimore, MD 21207
410-966-6823
*Certifies facilities that participate
in federal Medicare and Medicaid
programs. Determines whether
facilities meet required federal
standards.*

**Health Insurance Association
of America**
Fulfillment Department
1025 Connecticut Avenue, Suite
  1200
Washington, DC 20036
202-223-7780 800-942-4242
*Has pamphlets, brochures, and
instructions on a variety of health
insurances. Has hotline to answer
questions and respond to
complaints.*

**Health Resources and Services
Administration**
Health and Human Resources
  Department
5600 Fishers Lane
Rockville, MD 20857
301-443-2086 Information
*Supports state efforts to deliver
quality and cost-effective health care
to underserved areas.*

**Institute for Women's Policy
Research**
1400 20th Street, NW
Washington, DC 20036
202-785-5100
*Public-policy research
organization that focuses on
women's issues, including health
care and comprehensive family and
medical leave programs.*

Medical Information Bureau
P.O. Box 105
Essex Station
Boston, MA 02112
617-426-3660
*Consists of member insurance
organizations that keep records of
individual medical histories to
verify data on insurance
applications.*

**National Association of
Community Health Centers
#122**
1330 New Hampshire Avenue,
  NW
Washington, DC 20036
202-659-8008
*Provides the medically
underserved with health services.
Members include community health
centers and other community
health-care programs.*

National Coalition for Cancer Survivorship
323 Eighth Street
Albuquerque, NM 87102
505-764-9956
Organization of groups and individuals concerned with cancer survivorship. Can offer sources of support, advice, and legal aid for cancer patients and their families.

National Council Against Health Fraud Resource Center
P.O. Box 1747
Allentown, PA 18105
215-437-1795 800-821-6671
Focuses on educating women on health issues and health care fraud.

National Health Council
1730 M Street NW, #500
Washington, DC 20036
202-785-3913
Membership includes health agencies, businesses, insurance and government groups interested in health. Serves as an information clearinghouse on health careers.

National Institutes of Health
Health and Human Services
Department
9000 Rockville Pike
Bethesda, MD 20892
301-496-4000 301-496-2433
The Public Affairs Department can direct you to the appropriate professionals associated with breast cancer.

National Women's Health Network
1325 G Street, NW
Washington, DC 20005
202-347-2240
Acts as a clearinghouse on women's health issues; monitors federal health policies and legislation. Interested in breast cancer; provides information and referrals.

People for Health Insurance Equity
554 East 82nd Street
New York, NY 10028
212-535-7947
Involved in public advocacy to promote equality in the health-care industry, specifically as it relates to health insurance issues.

Public Health Service
Health and Human Services
Department
200 Independence Avenue SW
Washington, DC 20201
202-690-7163 Information
Advises the public on a variety of health issues. Develops health resources and establishes national health policy. Monitors U.S. health.

U.S. Health and Human Services Department
200 Independence Avenue, SW
Washington, DC 20201
800-336-4797 Information
202-690-6867
Directs activities of Public Health Service. Assists the public on a variety of health issues including costs and expenditures.

SECTION FOUR

Medical Associations and Boards

A list of medical boards and associations that in some instances can provide you with literature and reports on breast cancer. You can call to verify a physician's board certification.

American Association of Women Radiologists
1891 Preston White Drive
Reston, VA 22091
703-648-8900
Members are physicians involved in diagnostic or therapeutic radiology; maintains a resource center for current information for women.

American Board of Radiology
Suite 440
Birmingham, MI 48009
313-645-0600
Will verify radiologists and facilities.

American Board of Medical Specialties
10007 Church Street
Suite 404
Evanston, IL 60201
800-776-2378
Will verify a physicians's board certification.

American College of Obstetricians and Gynecologists
Resource Center
409 12th Street, SW
Washington, DC 20024
202-638-5577
Specializes in diseases of women; maintains a library of information.

American College of Physicians
Independence Mall West
6th Street at Race
Philadelphia, PA 19106
800-523-1546 215-351-2400
Membership includes physicians, internists, nonsurgical specialists. Monitors legislation and regulations relating to health policy.

American College of Radiology
1891 Preston White Drive
Reston, VA 22091
703-648-8900 800-227-5463
Publications
Professional society of certified radiologists who specialize in X ray, ultrasound, nuclear medicine, MRI for treatment of cancer; maintains a library of information.

American College of Surgeons
55 East Erie Street
Chicago, IL 60611
312-664-4050
Maintains a list of hospitals with approved breast programs. Will provide names of certified surgeons who specialize in breast surgery in your area.

American Council on Science and health
1995 Broadway, 2nd Fl.
New York, NY 10023
212-362-7044
Provides consumers with literature and reports on a variety of health issues. Involved with public health advocacy.

American Medical Association
515 North State Street
Chicago, IL 60610
800-621-8335 Information
312-464-5000
Has 54 state groups that monitor the medical industry and its assorted fields. Cooperates in setting standards for medical schools and hospitals. Publishes many journals.

American Medical Women's Association
801 North Fairfax Street, Suite 400
Alexandria, VA 22314
703-838-0500
Membership of female physicians. Has 160 local groups to lobby for improvement in women's health care; evaluates products for women's health. Promotes education programs.

American Society for Therapeutic Radiology and Oncology
1101 Market, 14th Floor
Philadelphia, PA 19107
215-574-3180
Member association of physicians who limit practice to radiology. Also includes members in supporting health care or radiology.

American Society of Clinical Oncology
435 North Michigan Avenue, Suite 1717
Chicago, IL 60611
312-644-0828
Will provide medical professionals with a directory of member oncologists in specific geographic locations.

American Society of Clinical Pathologists
1001 Pennsylvania Avenue, NW, #725
Washington, DC 20004
202-347-4450

*Membership includes
pathologists, physicians, registered
certified medical technologists, and
technicians. Monitors regulations
and research in pathology.*

**American Society of Internal
Medicine**
2011 Pennsylvania Avenue, NW,
　Suite 800
Washington, DC 20005
202-835-2746
*Professional society concerned
with social, economic, financial,
and political factors affecting health
care, cost reimbursement, and
insurance.*

**American Society of Plastic
and Reconstructive Surgeons**
444 East Algonquin Road
Arlington Heights, IL 60005
800-635-0635
708-228-9900 24 hr. patient
　referral
*Provides information on
reconstruction and will mail a list
of certified reconstructive surgeons
by geographic location.*

**College of American
Pathologists**
325 Waukegan Road
Publications
Northfield, IL 60093
708-446-8800

*Physicians practicing in
pathology or laboratory examination
of patients, conducts laboratory
accreditation program and
laboratory proficiency testing.
Pamphlets.*

**National Board of Medical
Examiners**
393 Chestnut Street
Philadelphia, PA 19104
215-590-9500
*Monitors the examination and
licensing through state agencies of
medical professionals; establishes
criteria for certification and
qualifications.*

National Medical Association
1012 10th Street, NW
Washington, DC 20001
202-347-1895
*Professional society of black
physicians. Conducts symposia and
workshops. Mailing list of
physicians by region.*

**Pharmaceutical Manufacturers
Association**
New Medicines in Development
1100 15th Street, NW
Washington, DC 20005
202-835-3400
*Results of testing new medicines
on cancer and information on
research of treatments.*

SECTION FIVE

. . . .

Other Sources

A listing of reference books that may be found in your local, county, state, or medical library.

American Federation of Clinical Oncologic Societies
Directory of Members
Published by the American Federation of Clinical Societies
This book list physicians who are members of several societies associated with the treatment of cancer. Memberships are board-certified with experience in cancer treatments. Members of the Society of Surgical Oncology are experienced in cancer surgery.

American Medical Directory
Directory of Physicians in the United States
535 North Dearborn Street
Chicago, IL 60610
Compiled and published by the AMA as a reference source of biographical and professional information on individual physicians in the U.S. Verified information supplied by physician, medical schools, and licensing agencies.

Directory of Medical Specialists
The Official American Board of Medical Specialties
Macmillan Directory Division
Wilmette, IL 60091
Published by Marquis Who's Who. Comprehensive listing of physicians certified by the 23 individual board of the ABMS. Current professional and biographical info. on certified physicians listed by state, city and town. Look for doctors with advanced training as cancer specialists or oncologists.

Directory of Physicians in the United States
33rd Edition 1992
American Medical Association
Division of Survey and Data Resources
A listing of members and nonmembers of the AMA obtained from physicians and verified by information by medical schools. Call 800-776-2378 to verify a physicians's certification.

225

Questionable Doctors Disciplined by States or the Federal Government
A Public Citizen Health
  Research Group Report
Ingrid Vantuinen/Phyllis
  McCarthy;/Sidney Wolfe, MD

Lists doctors disciplined for reasons such as substandard care, drug or alcohol abuse, criminal convictions, and misprescribing drugs.

Suggested Readings

Books

Berg, Karen, and John Bostwick III, M.D. *A Woman's Decision*. St. Louis: Mosby Publishing, 1984.

Brinker, Nancy, *The Race Is Run One Step at a Time*. New York: Simon and Schuster, 1990.

deMonlin, Daniel. *A Short History of Breast Cancer*. Dordrecht, Netherlands: Academic Publishers, 1983.

Greenberg, Mimi. *Invisible Scars*. New York: St. Martin's Press, 1988.

Gross, Amy, and Dee Ito, *Women Talk About Breast Surgery*. New York: Clarkson Potter, 1990.

Harris, Jay R., et al. *Breast Diseases, 2nd ed.* Philadelphia: J. B. Lippincott, 1991.

Hirshaut, Yashar, M.D., and Peter Pressman, M.D. *Breast Cancer: The Complete Guide*. New York: Bantam Books, 1992.

Inlander, Charles B., and Ed Weiner. *Take This Book to the Hospital with You*. Emmaus, Pa.: Rodale Press, 1985.

Kelly, Patricia, T. *Understanding Breast Cancer Risk*. Philadelphia: Temple University Press, 1991.

Love, Susan M., M.D. *Dr. Susan Love's Breast Book*. Boston: Addison-Wesley, 1990.

Mayer, Thomas R., and Gloria Gilbert Mayer. *The Health Insurance Alternative: A Complete Guide to Health Maintenance Organizations*. New York: Putnam Publishing Group, 1984.

Milan, Albert K., M.D. *Breast Self-Examination*. New York: Liberty Publishing/ Workman Publishing, 1980.

Naifeh, Steven, and Gregory White Smith, eds. *The Best Doctors in America*. Aiken, S.C.: Woodward/White, Inc., 1992.

Starer, Daniel. *Who Knows What*. New York: Henry Holt & Co., 1992.

Strax, Philip, M.D. *Make Sure You Do Not Have Breast Cancer*. New York: St. Martin's Press, 1991.

Williams, Stephen J., and Sandra J. Guerra. *A Consumer's Guide to Health Care Services*. New Jersey: New England Journal of Medicine/Prentice Hall, 1985.

Journals

"Cancer Statistics." *CA—A Cancer Journal for Clinicians*. American Cancer Society (January/February 1994).

Belchetz, P. E. "Drug Therapy: Hormonal Treatment of Post-Menopausal Women." *New England Journal of Medicine*, vol. 30, no. 12 (March 24, 1994).

Bondy, M. L., et al. "The Validation of Breast Cancer Risk Assessment Model in Women with a Positive Family History." *Journal of the National Cancer Institute*, vol. 86, no. 8 (April 20, 1994).

Harris, Russell. "Breast Cancer Among Women in Their Forties: Toward a Reasonable Research Agenda." *Journal of the National Cancer Institute*, vol. 86, no. 6 (March 16, 1994).

Olivotto, I. A. et al. "Adjuvant Systemic Therapy and Survival after Breast Cancer." *New England Journal of Medicine*, vol. 330, no. 2 (March 24, 1994).

Samet, J. M. et al. "Determinants of Receiving Breast Conserving Surgery." *Cancer: An Interdisciplinary International Journal of the American Cancer Society*, vol. 73, no. 9 (May 1, 1994).

Other

Cancer Facts and Figures—1994. American Cancer Society, Inc.

Chemotherapy and You. U.S. Dept. of Health and Human Services, Public Health Services, National Institutes of Health.

"Comparative Clinical and Financial Standards." *The DRG Handbook*. HCIA and Ernst & Young, 1993.

Hospital Inpatient Charges. HCIA, Inc. Ann Arbor, MI 1993.

Patient's Guide to Breast Cancer Treatment. Anne Moore, M.D., with Armand S. Cortese, M.D., and the New York Hospital Breast Cancer Tumor Board, New York Hospital—Cornell Medical Center.

Radiation Therapy and You. U.S. Dept of Health and Human Services, Public Health Services, National Institutes of Health.

"Profiles for Detailed Statistics." "Selected States and Practice Arrangements," *Physician's Marketplace Statistics*. American Medical Association.

Source Book of Health Insurance Data. Health Insurance Association of America (HIAA).

State Administrative Officials. The Council of State Governments, 1980–1990.

Taking Time. U.S. Dept. of Health and Human Services, Public Health Services, National Institutes of Health.

Washington Information Directory. Congressional Quarterly, 1993.

Index

Costs, 141–50
  biopsy, 50, 51, 52, 147, 148
  breast reconstruction, 123, 124,
    125, 148, 149
  CAT scan, 44, 147
  chart of, 147–50
  chemotherapy, 149
  DNA flow cytometry, 57, 150
  mammograms, 37, 41, 147, 149
  MRI, 43, 147
  nuclear scans, 147
  ultrasound, 42, 147
  see also Insurance
Credit cards, 23, 154
Cyclophosphamide, 115
Cysts, breast, 5, 30, 31–32, 49
Cytoxan, 115

D

Deodorants, 113
Depression (emotional), 127–28
Diet
  breast cancer diagnosis and, 138
  chemotherapy and, 117, 118
  hormone therapy and, 120
  as risk factor, 66–67
Diethylstilbestrol (DES) risk factor,
  64
Differentiation, 56
Directory of Medical Specialists, 80
DNA flow cytometry, 57, 150
Doctors. *See* Physicians; *specific
  specialities*
Doxorubicin (Adriamycin), 115
Drugs
  chemotherapeutic, 115, 117
  for chemotherapy-related nausea,
    117
  costs, 149, 150
  in hormone therapy, 119

E

Edema. *See* Arm swelling
EKG (electrocardiogram), 23, 26,
  52
  costs, 147, 150

Emotions
  as cancer risk factor, 66
  for coping with breast cancer,
    133–40
  diagnosis-related, 15, 61–62, 138
  postsurgery and treatments,
    127–28
  seeking help for, 128, 137
Environmental risk factors, 66
Estrogen, 65, 119, 120; *see also*
  Hormone therapy
Estrogen receptor assay (ERA), 17,
  56, 57, 119
Ethnic origin, as risk factor, 66
Exercise, 67, 120, 127, 138–39

F

Family doctor, 11, 19, 30
Family medical history, 4, 18, 31, 63,
  71, 104
Family support, 135–36
Fibrocystic breast changes, 5, 30,
  31–32, 65
Finances. *See* Costs; Insurance
5-fluorouracil (5-FU), 115
Food and Drug Administration, 35,
  36, 39, 46
Frozen section analysis, 14–15, 17,
  51, 55, 150

G

Group therapy, 21, 137
Guilt feelings, 61–62, 138
Gynecologists, 11, 19, 30, 147

H

Hair loss, 116–17
Health insurance. *See* Insurance
Heart disease, 121
HMO (Health Maintenance
  Organization)
  breast center coverage, 95
  hospital coverage, 90
  mammography, 37
  second opinions, 19, 78